One Lump, or Two?
My Personal *Breast Cancer* Journey

By Linda Sadler

Published by Rochester Media
Edited by Sarah L. Hovis
www.RochesterMedia.com

Book design by Beth Lee
Cover photography by Liz Gibbons
Back cover portrait by Peggy Wilke

# Dedication

This journal is dedicated to my husband of over 40 years, Michael, my daughter, Melanie, and my son, Chad, all of whom I love very, very much.

I am grateful to my friend of many years, Nancy Grimmer, who when hearing of my diagnosis immediately told me that she was right beside me — that I wasn't going through this alone.

Also appreciated, are the family members, friends, and prayer warriors of friends that have lent me their love, support, kindness, offers of favors, and who continue to help me through this journey. Including Sarah Hovis, who edited and formatted this book.

My "A-Team" of doctors: Dr. Manisha Kia, my primary care physician; Dr. Linsey Gold, my cancer surgeon; Dr. Kimberly Pummill, my plastic surgeon; and Dr. Rizwan Danish, my oncologist.

The love of the *One* who made me, my Saviour and Lord, who guided the surgeons and doctors and strengthened me throughout this. His love makes me whole and to Him be all the glory.

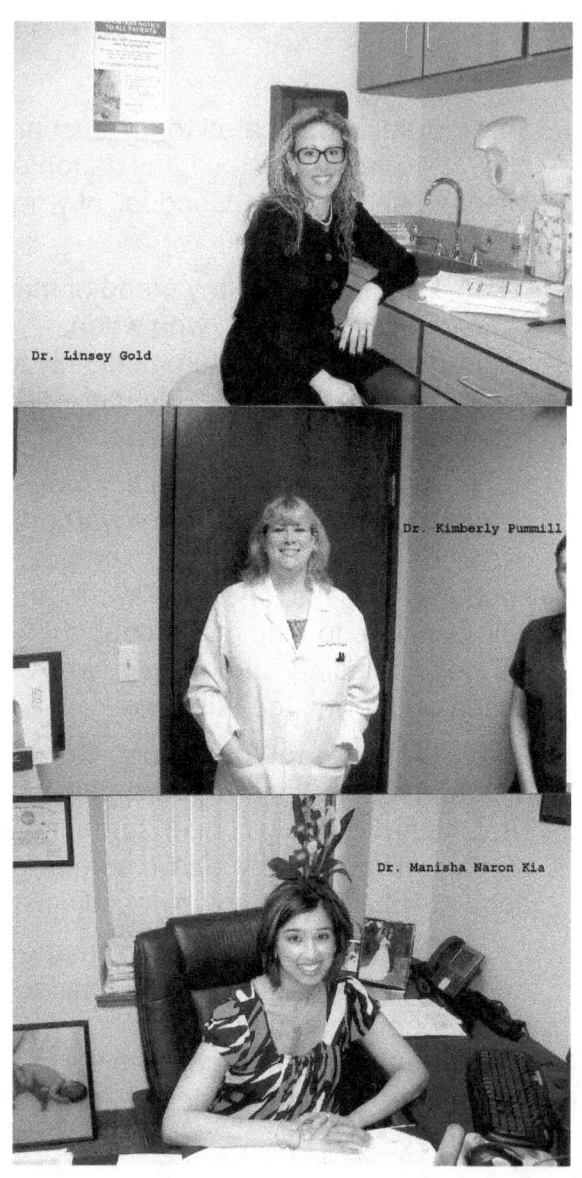

Dr. Linsey Gold

Dr. Kimberly Pummill

Dr. Manisha Naron Kia

# Contents

My journey began on August 18, 2009, when I received news of my pathology report from my doctor.

Before I get ahead of myself, let me begin the story by telling you that in July 2009, I had my regular physical and was given a clean bill of health. I asked my doctor, Dr. Manisha Kia, if I should proceed with my regular mammogram, or if I could skip it this time. I was instructed to go.

A week after the first mammogram the radiology department called me. I was told that they needed to take more views, and that I should come in again. At the time I thought, *How odd. I've never had to do this before.*

I went, however, and had a second mammogram. Then I was told I would also be having a digital mammography as well as a sonogram. Again, I was thinking to myself, *This is not normal*, but went along.

During the sonogram, attention kept being directed to the left side (near the milk duct) of my left breast. I kept asking questions as to whether they saw something, or if there was something wrong, but I was only told that the radiologist was with another patient, and that she would talk to me shortly. It was at that time I asked for my husband to be brought into the room, as I needed to feel his hand in mine for support.

When he entered, he asked what was wrong, and I told him I didn't know, but that I did not have a good feeling about this.

The radiologist was still not available when I dressed, so I asked the technician if I could just go home. She said, "Yes," and I was then told that the results would be available within three to five business days. That time crept by, but the next Tuesday I was called by my doctor's office and explained that a needle biopsy would be required.

That appointment was made and for the next several days I had trouble sleeping, relaxing my mind, and just feeling normal. Anxiety took over and I finally called my doctor and asked if I could be given a light sedative to relax me before the test. She called in the prescription and I took the pill one hour before my test.

The day of the needle biopsy, my husband was not able to go with me, so my son Chad dropped me off and my daughter Melanie met me at the radiology office. When she first saw me in the dressing room, she asked, "Mom. Are you on drugs? You look loopy."

I told her I'd been given a light sedative, but I didn't care how I looked; I just wanted to get through the test.

The attendants who took care of me were very kind and gentle, helping me into a surgical gown and then leading me into an examining room. There, I was placed facedown on a long table that had a large opening, extending down through it. My left breast was placed into the hole and the machine immediately started to compress against it.

Instant pain developed, and I remember tears welling up in my eyes. I told the attendant that I was really hurting and they backed off the machine a little, repositioned me, and proceeded once again.

The doctor that actually gave me the injections (two in each breast) comforted me and told me that I was doing just fine and explained every step that would be taken.

The injections were given with some discomfort and stinging because the second one had to be given deeper so that the whole breast was numb.

After the numbing, a small slit was made and the computerized machine did some constant clicking, taking several samples. The left breast was given a pressure bandage and it was off to do the right breast. After more samples were taken on the right side, the test was finally complete and I was allowed to dress.

After changing back into my clothes, the two assistants handed me a pink rose with baby's breath. Little did I know how significant that pink rose would become for me in the future.

I was told that within five to seven days my doctor would have the results of the needle biopsy, and that she would call me with the results.

Sure enough, on the morning of August 18, 2009, I received a call from Dr. Kia asking me to come into her office at 11:00 a.m. Luckily, my wonderful and supportive husband drove me there.

I remember thinking to myself, *Take deep breathes Linda. Now blow out. Take another deep breath, and now blow it out.*

When we arrived in the waiting room, it seemed like it was hours before my name was called, but actually it was only 15 to 20 minutes. I had a dream the night before I was to see Dr. Kia. I dreamt that my son Chad went with me to the doctor's office and Dr. Kia was sitting on the stool at the end of the examining table with an electric razor in her hand. She handed the razor to Chad and asked him to shave her head.

I think I realized at that moment that God was telling me that I had cancer and that this was a journey I had to take. I shared this dream with Dr. Kia and she asked me how she looked bald.

I told her she was still cute, and we both shared a laugh. Then came the more serious conversation.

Dr. Kia told me she had come to talk with me one-on-one, regardless of whether the news was good or bad. Her next words to me were, "Linda, you did everything right. You had your physical and you had your mammogram like you faithfully do every year, but the pathology report from the needle biopsy shows cancer in both breasts."

At that moment, I remember just feeling numb. *Cancer* in both breasts — how?

I just had a physical and was fine, and my mammogram from the year before showed nothing. Dr. Kia saw the tears beginning, and she told me I would be fine. That it was discovered early, and from what she had seen in the report, the cancer was confined.

Her next statement was that she wanted me to go to the surgeon's office the very next day at 8:00 a.m.

I remember leaving Dr. Kia's office and returning to the waiting room, and seeing my patient husband.

My face must have told him immediately that something was wrong.

I waited until we were walking to the car, with his hand in mine, and I gave him the news. He was completely stunned, but he also reassured me that we should hope for the best.

On the drive home, I dreaded having to tell my children. As soon as I got home, I walked upstairs to where my son Chad was working on the computer.

Chad asked immediately, "What's up mom?"

I gulped, took a deep breath, and the words, "I have breast cancer in both breasts," blurted out of my mouth.

At that moment, the reality fully set in and I sobbed uncontrollably. I remember thinking, *I can't breathe. I can't breathe*, as the tears just flowed. I stumbled into the bathroom and grabbed a towel, trying to muffle my sobs.

After the tears finally subsided, I immediately called my daughter, Melanie. When I reached her on the phone, I told her that my test results came back, and I had cancer in both breasts.

A, "Wow, mom. How could this have happened?" came out of her mouth. In the next instant, this take charge, authoritative voice told me not to worry. That she would call the insurance company to see what would be covered, that she would find me a surgeon, and that I needed to go to the University of Michigan Hospital in Ann Arbor, Michigan.

I told her, "I don't want your father to have to drive from Grand Blanc to Ann Arbor to see me."

"Mom. You have cancer. This is nothing to mess with."

Her assertiveness was a pleasant surprise to me, as she can often be elusive and seemingly uncaring.

I explained to Melanie that my appointment with the surgeon was at 8:00 a.m. the following day, and I wanted to keep it. I had faith in Dr. Kia's judgment, and I wanted to show her that by seeing the surgeon she suggested.

Wednesday, August 19. Mike was not available to drive me to the surgeon, so Chad willingly took me. As is their standard policy when seeing a new patient, I was given two pages of family history and personal information to fill out, along with being asked for my ID and insurance card. Again, the wait seemed forever, but I am sure it was no more than 15 or 20 minutes.

I remember being extremely nervous before I was called to the inner office area, but when they finally said my name, I entered a very patient-friendly hallway with '50s-styled hats hanging on the walls. Then I turned into a room with a lovely green and pink quilt hanging on the wall, along with the usual examining table and instrumentation that appear in every doctor's office.

There was a knock on the door, and in came this tiny-framed woman — Dr. Linsey Gold — who looked young enough to be my daughter.

She extended her hand to mine, and the first words that came out of her mouth were, "Linda, you're going to be all right. You're going to be all right." Her next words were, "Welcome to Boobs-R-Us!"

I remember chuckling with her and immediately some of my fear disappeared.

She then proceeded to examine my bruised and sore breasts and another sonogram was performed. Afterwards, I dressed and followed her into the consultation room.

We went over the pathology report together and I was told that she felt very confident the cancer was contained in both breasts. I then told her that I didn't care if I was operated on the very next day and both breasts were removed. I just wanted this to be over.

Her reply was, "Why would you do something so drastic when I don't really believe it is necessary?" Again, more of my fear melted away and the consultation continued.

The cancer in the right breast is called high-grade duct carcinoma with only a 5-10% of the specimen affected by cancer. The left breast was also stage one, possibly stage two, and is known as infiltrating duct carcinoma. Surgery would be required on both sides.

I was also told that before surgery, a Magnetic Resonance Imaging (MRI) test was necessary to determine the actual size of each tumor, and to see if there are any "hot spots" that were not picked up in the proceeding tests.

As I waited for my MRI to begin, Dr. Gold told me that during my surgery, three to four node biopsy samples would be taken to make sure the cancer had not infiltrated the lymph nodes. If those were clear, then the only procedure would be the lumpectomy. If those biopsy samples came back positive, I would be taken back into surgery within two days (it takes that long for the pathology reports to return).

If I needed chemotherapy, it would be a Monday through Friday procedure, for seven weeks of radiation on the right breast, and then a Monday through Friday procedure for another seven weeks on the left breast.

The treatment would take place in Clarkston, Michigan and require driving back and forth 28 miles roundtrip every day.

And so, I prepared myself as much as I could for my cancer journey to get into full swing within the next couple of weeks.

Friends, family, and loved ones have already been a source of great hope, courage, strength, and love to me. I will continue to journal through all the stages of this disease and draw on the strength of others and the Lord who loves me so. I do not know what my future holds, but I know the *One* who holds my future. I know there is a reason that I have been given this challenge, but my prayer is that God will be glorified through it all and maybe, just maybe, I can be an encouragement to someone else taking this same journey.

_August_

It is Monday, August 24, 2009, and I am
on to the next trek of this journey. I just
received a call from Dr. Gold's office (my
surgeon) and my MRI is scheduled for
Thursday, August 27 at 7:00 p.m. Fifteen
minutes later, I received a call from Dr.
Kia that an Echo Cardiogram (EKG) is
necessary for medical clearance before
surgery, and that appointment will be
August 26 at 4:00 p.m.

It looks like it is all systems go.
Things are starting to progress rather
rapidly now.

It's Tuesday, August 25, and Dr.
Gold's office requested that I meet with
the radiologist/oncologist that will be
performing my radiation treatments after
my surgery. This appointment is in
Clarkston and set for Thursday,
September 3, 2009 at 9:30 a.m.

I was also told today that I would
need to have genetic testing done. This
is probably to see if I am pre-disposed to
any other major diseases because of
family history.

On my mother's side of the family there is heart disease, diabetes, Alzheimer's, and Parkinson's disease. I don't know much about my father's side, as both grandparents died at young ages. The only information I know for sure is that my grandfather was French Canadian, and my grandmother was Irish.

Boy. The phone is ringing off the hook these days.

It is still Tuesday afternoon, 12:37 p.m., and my surgeon's office wants me to go at 1:15 p.m. today for the genetic testing. Since the test is sent to Utah, it takes two to three weeks for the results to come in.

I arrived at Dr. Gold's office and was given the test kit and taken to the lab area. The entire test didn't take more than 15 minutes.

First, I was given a very small bottle of Scope mouthwash and asked to swish a small cupful around in my mouth for 30 seconds. Next, I was instructed to spit the contents from my mouth into a sterile container and then repeat the same steps one more time. Then I was told to take my tongue and roll it around my teeth and on both sides of my cheek area and spit my saliva (sounds gross, I know) into the sterile container twice.

Test over, and I am on my way to the next test tomorrow. One step closer to the pre-surgery appointment where the actual surgery date will be determined.

Today is Wednesday, August 26, 2009, and it seems like almost every day God encourages me and strengthens me with word that I have been prayed for by someone else, or I have been added to another church's prayer list. Yesterday my daughter Melanie called me to say that she has reconnected with an old high school friend, Roger Carlson.

Roger is now a pastor and has started praying for me personally, along with his church congregation.

My twin sisters-in-law, Juanita and Anita, have both told me they have also put in requests for prayer on my behalf at their churches. An old friend at Bethany Baptist is praying for me, and two other friends, Joyce and John Hovis, have placed me on their church's prayer list as well. It goes on and on. I am continually amazed at the kindness of people that I don't even know and have never met formally. What a blessing!

When I was coming out of the lab on Tuesday, August 25 after having the genetic test, I noticed in the atrium beautiful pink zinnias for sale. Of course knowing me, I had to stop and admire them. Standing there was a young lady with her mother, father, and her brother. I made the comment that pink was the color for breast cancer awareness.

"Oh, I know," she said. "I walk each year for the cancer cause."

I thanked her and proceeded to tell her that she was walking for me now, as I had just recently been diagnosed. She then said, "I'm sorry. I'll be sure to walk even more now."

Imagine. Someone I casually meet in a hospital area giving me encouragement and support.

*Thank you Lord for your goodness. I feel like I am not alone in this fight. I appreciate your love for me.*

Later today I go for my EKG, and then tomorrow evening, it is on to my MRI.

Updates to come.

Today is Thursday morning, August 27, the day of my MRI. I guess I will really need to push drinking water today so that my veins are nice and plump. It's my understanding that I will have pictures taken in the MRI machine. Then, I will have an IV placed into my arm, where dye will be introduced into my veins.

I will probably be asked to wait for a while, and then be placed back into the machine for more pictures. The whole process should take about an hour, but knowing how my little veins sometimes give the doctors trouble, we will see.

The EKG on August 26 ended up being the easiest test I've had to date. By the time the nurse got me all hooked up with the receptors (I guess that's what they are called) and turned on the machine, the test seemed to be over in two minutes. The report is my "ticker" is fine with no apparent abnormalities.

Phew! That's a relief.

So, now it's time to drink lots of water today, and I will report on how the MRI went after its completion.

It turns out having a MRI isn't so bad, just really noisy.

Upon arriving for my appointment I had to — you guessed it — fill out paperwork again.

Don't you just love it?

You would think the records would be transferred from one office to another, but I guess each office has its own recordkeeping system in the computer.

Anyway, once the papers were filled out, I was led into a dressing room and asked to put on one of those beautiful blue gowns that opens in the front. The assistant went over the procedure, and an IV was started. Honestly, I did a lot better than I thought I would.

Immediately, I was taken into the imaging room and placed facedown on a table with two holes in the bottom where my breasts hung down in all their glory.

My face was placed into a foam-like mold with a mirror in the bottom, but I kept my eyes closed during the whole test. The machine pulled me into position and then without warning a loud alarm-like noise started. It reminded me of the fire alarm signals we had when I was in elementary school. The next noise I heard was a very loud *buzz, buzz, buzz*, and then a deeper toned *bang, bang, bang.*

Thank goodness for the earplugs they gave me.

Just when you think you can't stand the sound any longer, it is quiet and then the buzzing and banging start up again. All in all, I was only there a total of 45 minutes. The only hitch was that the mammography X-rays were not given to me, nor the records from the same, so tomorrow morning I must call Dr. Gold's office and request that they be sent, or picked up by me and taken to the MRI location.

One more test down... yeah!

It is Friday morning, August 28, and I have been on the phone since 8:00 a.m. It seems that yesterday I needed to take my previous mammograms records from up to seven years ago, as well as my recent breast ultrasound records with me when I went to the MRI location — oops!

The nurse in Dr. Gold's office apologized. She is relatively new in the office and thankfully she said she would take full responsibility for the glitch.

My main problem is that I had my first mammograms in Grand Blanc at McLaren Imaging Center, and the most recent images have been taken at Genesys Diagnostic Imaging. So, it looks like I will be running from office-to-office unless they have couriers that can assist me.

Update: After several phone calls, my records from McLaren Imaging will be ready for me to pick after 1:00 p.m. today, and a courier will send the records from Genesys Diagnostic Imaging to both Dr. Gold's office and the MRI location. Phew. What a relief.

Today is Sunday, August 30, 2009. This is the first day in a while that I haven't had to go in for any testing or run around to pick up X-rays, etc. It feels good just to be able to sit and relax.

The original X-rays that were taken at Genesys Diagnostics will be delivered by courier this morning to the MRI location on Lennon Road. After the MRI reports are completed and the size determined on the tumors, I'm sure Dr. Gold will call me in for consult once again, and hopefully, my surgery date will be finalized.

It is now Monday morning, August 31, 2009, and I just made a second phone call to the radiology office to make sure that the X-ray and sonogram reports were delivered. As we suspected, some of the bills for our co-pay amounts are starting to arrive for payment. Guess we better get used to that fact. At least our yearly deductible for a married couple has not yet been met.

Poor Mike. I know he is worried about my health, and now we have extra doctor bills to cope with. Just have to take it day at a time — and one bill at a time.

It is Tuesday, September 1, 2009 already. So much for relaxing. Word just came from my surgeon, Dr. Gold that the genetic testing I had last Tuesday has to be redone. Evidently, not enough cells were retrieved to complete it, So, I'm off to the Genesys Hospital lab again today at 2:30 p.m. It is a simple test, so no big deal. And I was assured that I would not be charged this time.

Ok. That test is over. Evidently DNA use to be retrieved by a blood test, but the new test is done with mouthwash swished around in the mouth and spit into a sterile container, which means it's supposed to be simpler. The only problem that I can see is that because of its newness, not everyone is administering it the same way.

The first lab technician had me swish the Scope around in my mouth two times for 30 seconds each time and then had me bring up saliva and spit into the container. The second lab technician had me swish for a full minute two times, and then bring up saliva. Hopefully, we have enough good cells to test this time.

I feel like a guinea pig, but it is important testing for gathering information for myself, as well as the surgeons; it will tell me what I might also be genetically pre-disposed to.

I also found out when I was at Dr. Gold's office today, that the MRI I had on Thursday takes about three to four days for completion. I'm hoping that means I will have the results sometime later this week, and bring me one step closer to my surgery date.

I have been trying to keep myself busy with working on my father's back porch (Mike and I mixed, poured, and spread 22 bags of cement) as the old porch was deteriorating badly. We also built him a 10' x 12' deck on the front of his house this summer. Mike's parents also needed a deck on the back of their house for the same reason, so Mike, Chad, and I also tackled that job. It felt good to be able to help out both parents. So between the deck projects, the staining of our own deck, and my journaling, I am managing to keep my mind occupied.

Had a busy morning watering my flowers, making blueberry pancakes (at my husband's request) did morning dishes, made a pot of chili, and washed a load of dirty clothes.

Now, all of a sudden, it's like God is saying to me, "Linda, sit down and reflect." Bible verses were running through my head, giving me strength and comfort. Please let me share them:

*I have loved thee with an everlasting love.*
Jeremiah 31:3

*Rest in the Lord, and wait patiently for him.*
Psalm 37:7

*Thou wilt keep him in perfect peace, whose mind is stayed on thee.*
Isaiah 26:3

*God hath not given us a spirit of fear; but of power, and of love, and of sound mind.*
2 Timothy 1:7

*Cast they burdens upon the Lord, and he shall sustain thee.*
Psalm 55: 22

*The Lord is my shepherd,*
*I shall not want.*

Psalm 23:1

*God is our refuge and strength, a very*
*present help in trouble.*

Psalm 46:1

*What time I am afraid, I will trust in thee.*

Psalm 56:3

*Wait on the Lord, be of good courage,*
*and he shall strengthen thine heart; wait,*
*I say on the Lord.*

Psalm 27:14

*But they that wait upon the Lord shall*
*renew their strength; they shall mount up*
*with wings as eagles; they shall run, and*
*not be weary; and they shall walk,*
*and not faint.*

Isaiah 40:31

*Thank you Lord for your Word.*

Today is Thursday, September 3, 2009, and I just returned home from meeting with the radiologist/oncologist in the Clarkston office.

Dr. Miller was very kind and explained the radiation process to me. I was also examined and was told that the tumor in the right breast was approximately one centimeter, while the mass in the left breast was approximately two centimeters.

After the actual physical examination of the breasts, Dr. Miller called the MRI location on Lennon Road and talked to the doctors there — more bad news. The mass on the left breast has three small satellite tumors. The two at the top of that breast seem to be small, while the one near the lower part of the breast seems to be somewhat larger. Since they are not sure if these tumors are benign or malignant, I have to have another needle biopsy.

There is a good possibility that we may not be able to save enough tissue in the left breast to make it cosmetically pleasing, so it may have to be removed totally. We are also trying to see if the genetic test can somehow be rushed; it is important that we know if I am predisposed to cancer on my father's side of the family. I need to have as much background information as possible to make a well-informed decision.

I was asked to call my surgeon, Dr. Gold and talk to her regarding this information. She was with another patient when I called, and I was told she would call me back as soon as possible.

Today I just feel like shutting myself off from the outside world and hiding away in a cocoon. I just want this all to be over. I want to be well and whole again. I have taken every test that I was asked to, and I am tired of being probed and prodded.

*LORD, PLEASE GIVE ME THE STRENGTH TO ENDURE THIS TEST.*

It is Friday morning, September 4, 2009, and I received a phone call from Dr. Gold last night. She asked me not to be too upset over the results from the MRI.

She explained that even though it is an excellent diagnostic tool for determining exact locations, and size of tumors, that there are a lot of "false positive" reports. These false positives have caused many women like myself to say, "Enough already" and led them to make the decision of having radical surgery. These "hot spots" as they are called, don't always turn out to be cancer. We can't assume *anything* until another needle biopsy gives us more information.

Dr. Gold also told me that the radiologist uses different language when they read these reports, but that she speaks to them personally and feels that even though they say satellite tumors, the only way to really know what is in the tissue is to have another needle core biopsy test. Oh joy; just what I wanted to hear.

The larger, two-centimeter tumor in the lower quadrant is the one she is most concerned with. If that tumor is determined to be malignant, then she agrees a radical mastectomy would be required.

Yesterday I was ready to tell Dr. Gold, "Just take me in and remove both breasts."

I just want to be rid of this cancer, but today I realize that I don't want to be left with the "what ifs." *What if* I would have just had one more test. *What if* it is not malignant and we could have saved the left breast. What a roller coaster ride this journey has become.

I meet with Dr. Gold again on Tuesday, September 8, and she wants to give me the names of two plastic surgeons. One of the doctors is a male from Flint and the other is Dr. Kimberly Pummill from Grand Blanc. I guess if reconstructive surgery is necessary, she wants me to have met the plastic surgeon beforehand and discuss the different reconstructive options.

I am really confident in Dr. Gold and I trust her judgment. I feel very lucky to have such a wonderful, caring, and capable physician.

I received two cards in the mail this week. One from neighbors that said they were praying for me, and one from my sister-in-law, expressing the same sentiments. People don't realize how much encouragement these cards are to me. I think I have a better understanding now of what mail call means to our troops.

Those letters they receive must really boost their morale and make them realize how much they are loved and thought about at home.

Anyway, it was really comforting to me to receive these cards.

It is Saturday, the second day of the long Labor Day weekend, and even though Mike, my dad, and I were able to relax and take a ride this afternoon and visit the *Past Tense Country Store* in Lapeer, Michigan (dad purchased a breast cancer pin there for me to wear) my mind still reverts back to my cancer and needle biopsy that is ahead of me again.

They say knowledge is power, so I guess the more information I receive from these tests, the more capable I will be of making the right decision, and I know Dr. Gold wants me to take an active part in the decisions that are made regarding the upcoming procedures.

Here's to the rest of the long weekend with my family. These times mean so much to me.

It is Tuesday, September 8, 2009, and Labor Day weekend has ended. The first day of school was today, and I was back in Dr. Gold's office. She asked me what I had decided over the weekend regarding another needle biopsy, and I told her to go ahead and schedule it. I need to know for sure what is in the two-centimeter mass in the lower quadrant of my left breast.

If that mass turns out to be malignant, then we know for sure we cannot save the breast. The MRI-generated needle biopsy is scheduled for this week on Thursday, September 10, at 3:00 p.m. at the same location where the MRI was performed. I am also scheduled to see the plastic surgeon this Friday, September 11, at 2:15 p.m.

I decided to go with Dr. Pummill because she's local, female, and works on a regular basis with Dr. Gold, whom I really trust. Dr. Pummill will discuss my options directly related to the results from the needle biopsy, and I'm sure she will also go over reconstructive surgery if it is necessary.

Dr. Gold gave me a tentative surgery date of September 18, 2009 (exactly one month from my diagnosis) or September 22. The final date will be determined by the availability of the plastic surgeon and Dr. Gold, of course.

It seems like this journey has been longer than one month since I was diagnosed, but I know by the calendar it has not. The norm for surgery, I guess is typically one month from the original diagnosis. It seems that some cancers grow quickly, so a speedy surgery is usually done.

It is onward and upward with these next appointments, and then waiting two to three days again for the results from the biopsy.

Today is Wednesday, September 9, 2009, and I received my instructions for the MRI-guided needle biopsy tomorrow: nothing by mouth two hours prior to the test, wash the breast area with anti-bacterial soap, shave underarms (no deodorant) and wear a tight-fitting sports bra.

The sports bra is a scream!

I tried to put it on over my head and it got caught on my shoulder in a knot. I pulled and tugged, until I got it to cover the left breast and then had to reach my right arm behind my back to grab the bottom of the bra, so that I could pull it down in its correct position to cover the entire right breast.

I've never had so much trouble covering my boobs in my life! I can hardly wait to try this again tomorrow after I have the procedure when I am numb and bandaged. I'll probably need someone to help me. If it weren't X-rated, this would be a good video for *America's Funniest Home Videos*.

Oh well, at least in this whole process, there is something to chuckle about. Tomorrow at 3:00 p.m. I will have the final test — can't wait to get it over with. The technician called me last night to explain that I will be lying on my tummy again while the machine locates the mass.

Then comes the local injection, and then the deeper injection. After that, I shouldn't feel anything. The machine then proceeds to the area where the mass is located and removes the core sample. Pressure is applied to the wound and another mammogram is required to make sure that there is no blood pooling inside the breast.

Finally, it's get dressed, go home… and wait.

I think the hardest part of this whole journey is the waiting and the anticipation about the results from these tests. I guess that is where my faith has helped, "Trust in the Lord with all thine heart, and he will renew your strength."

*Thank you Lord for your love and your words of comfort.*

It is Thursday morning, September 10, 2009, and I took the first sports bra that I purchased back to the store and exchanged it for one that actually has a closure in the back. I just couldn't see myself struggling to get the original one over my head and on properly after the needle biopsy. Ouch!

Last night was a long night with much tossing and turning. My poor husband. I decided sometime after 2:40 a.m. to move to another room so I wouldn't disturb his sleep. It seemed my body was tired, but my mind just would not shut down. I kept thinking of the procedure that I would have to endure again. I am just not one of those people who can put things up on a shelf and forget about them completely.

Oh, how I wish I could.

Anyway, it is on to the final test this afternoon at 3:00 p.m. My next-door neighbor, Nancy Grimmer, will be going with me for moral support. Mike has to work today at the auto auction, my daughter is at her job, and my son also has a prior commitment. I'm glad they all have things to do to keep their minds busy. It helps them not to worry about me so much.

It is now 7:00 p.m., and I just arrived home from the MRI-guided needle biopsy. This one didn't go as well as the first biopsy. When I first arrived, Lisa, my technician, described the procedure to me again, and then an IV was started in my arm. I waited for what seemed a half hour or so before I was even taken into the procedure room. I was again placed face down on the table with my breasts hanging through the holes and was drawn into the MRI machine.

Again, the loud *buzzing* and *banging* noise filled the room. I was in the machine for several pictures to locate the area in question, and then dye was placed in the IV so that it would react to the tissue. Then more pictures were taken.

This whole process took one hour, and I almost didn't think I could stand being in the machine another minute. I was again numbed with two shots placed in the breast and then the MRI machine made a slight incision and eight to ten core samples were taken. This is when I started to sweat and got sick to my stomach. I started to feel like I had to get out of the machine *right now*.

Dr. Taha (who was administering the MRI) talked to me and asked if I was all right, while Lisa, the technician was rubbing my back and talking to me. I asked if the fan could be turned on higher so that I could get a little more cool air on my head. That seemed to help.

I then was pulled out of the machine, turned onto my back, and pressure was applied to the wound for 10 to 15 minutes. After that time had passed, a bandage of what they call "steri strips" was placed around the wound with a 4" x 4" pad and I was given some grape juice.

I think my sugar was a little low because I felt very shaky (I hadn't eaten anything since noon). After I finished the grape juice, I was taken into the mammogram room for two more views of the breast on which the biopsy had just been performed.

The mammogram was to ensure that no excess blood was still in the wound and that all the tissue samples were taken from the right area. I was told that the pathology report probably wouldn't be available until Tuesday or Wednesday of next week. So, the waiting game continues.

All in all, they said I did real well, but I am really, really glad that this is the last needle biopsy. Tomorrow afternoon I meet with the plastic surgeon and begin exploring my options.

I have only been home about 15 minutes, and Nancy, who went with me today, just brought me a dozen yellow roses tipped in orange, and a lovely card. What a nice gesture. We were also able to have dinner together after the procedure today. It is so nice to relax and chat after all the events of the day.

It is 12:15 in the morning, and I can't sleep. I am so sore to the touch that even the ice pack and the extra-strength Tylenol aren't making me any more comfortable. It feels like they went deeper into the breast for sample tissue this time, or they took out quite a few samples, because I am really hurting. I hope I don't have to be examined by the plastic surgeon today. Well, back to bed to try and get some rest.

It is Friday afternoon at 11:00 a.m., and I just received a call from my surgeon, Dr. Gold, who is on the way to her office. My genetic testing results came in, and it showed that I am at a 50% plus higher risk range for breast cancer and ovarian cancer, than the general public. It seems that this is on my father's side of the genetic tree. My decision became much easier after this information: I have decided to have a double mastectomy.

And later down the road, if Dr. Gold feels it necessary, I'll have a hysterectomy to remove my ovaries. I am also at a high-risk level for this type of cancer. All this because of a few genes. I am relieved. I feel free knowing that the cancer will be gone with the removal of both breasts.

I immediately called my brother, because he has a daughter. I felt they needed to know the genetic results. It also will affect my brothers, as they get older, as they will need to be tested for prostate cancer. I also notified my other niece Erin, because her dad (my older brother) is also in the genetic pool. Erin is also the mother of a new baby daughter. It is amazing how one little gene can affect so many lives.

Now when I go to meet with the plastic surgeon, Dr. Pummill, I will need to determine the type of implant and the size of the implant I want. My guys think I should go a little larger. Men. Go figure, right? My daughter agrees, and says that at least I won't have to worry about sagging and drooping as I age.

Everyone seems to have a sense of humor about this, and it really does help. I'll let my doctor determine the size according to my body proportions. I don't want to look too top heavy.

I met with Dr. Kimberly Pummill today, and my friend Nancy was there in the waiting room when I arrived. She told me she would not leave and be right there when the doctor finished with me.

Dr. Pummill explained two procedures: the first was a 10-hour surgery where tummy muscles were removed and used in the reconstruction process (I think this is called a flap surgery). I opted out of this procedure because of the time element. She told me this surgery could make me susceptible to a hernia and/or some instability with some coordination.

The second option is the one I chose. It is called tissue expander placement. A temporary expander sack is placed behind the muscle and is filled with a specific amount of saline over a period of several weeks. The tissue expanders stretch the skin allowing it to house the permanent implants.

Measurements were taken of both breasts as well as photos. I was told that I would get a lifetime guarantee with my new boobs. If anything happens, as far as movement of the implant or any type of damage, my insurance will pay for

49

another surgery. I now know that my surgery will take place next Tuesday, September 15, but I do not know the exact time yet. The hospital or the plastic surgeon's office will contact me.

The reason for moving up my surgery was twofold: Dr. Pummill will be out of town on September 23, so she did not want to perform the surgery on the 22, and then not be there the next day to make sure I was all right. Also, Dr. Gold, my other surgeon, could not be there on Friday, September 18, so a compromise date of September 15 was decided. Anyway, no more waiting. Now it is just surgery time and then the healing process begins.

It will be a real relief to have this all behind me, but I am confident that I have an exceptional team of female doctors that will take excellent care of me.

Today is Saturday, September 12, 2009; went to my mother-in-law's to celebrate her birthday (which was actually on the 9$^{th}$) with my dad, Mike, my two sisters-in-law, and of course, my father-in-law. We had a nice lunch and chit chatted for a while with everyone.

My father-in-law is usually not very verbal about things, but he gave me a hug and told me to keep a positive attitude. That really surprised me, but it was a sweet sentiment. Both sisters-in-law also gave me hugs and told me I am in their prayers. And of course, my wonderful mother-in-law told me she has been praying for me since the start of this journey and I would be in her prayers Tuesday morning.

It is such a blessing to have the support of a wonderful family and in-laws. It was also very nice to take a long, relaxing ride with my husband today. The weather was perfect, and so was the company. We really enjoy our weekends together.

Just two more days until my surgery and I am trying to stay upbeat and positive. Tomorrow, Sunday, I will be going with my daughter Melanie to a baby shower for the daughter of an old and dear friend. She is expecting her first child (a little girl) in November near my birthday. It will be really nice to see old friends again and to have some fun.

I am really looking forward to the healing process and the end of my cancer journey, and the start of a new journey of the rest of my life.

I feel a sense of freedom knowing that the cancer will be gone. Even though this has been a scary, difficult and sometimes painful process, I am very thankful for a wonderful doctor (Dr. Kia), a gifted surgeon (Dr. Gold) with a great sense of humor, and a skilled plastic surgeon (Dr. Pummill) whom I hear only good reports about. I know I am in good hands.

It is Monday morning, September 14, 2:22 a.m., and I am wide-awake. Can't sleep. I guess the anticipation of what is going to take place tomorrow is keeping me awake. I'm not really scared, but I am really nervous about how I will look and feel after surgery; I don't do very well with pain. I know from what my doctor said though, that I will not be allowed to suffer.

I know my guys here at home, are capable of taking care of themselves, but I really enjoy doing things for them: preparing their meals, doing the laundry, keeping the house clean and neat, mowing the lawn, and taking care of the dogs.

Had a very enjoyable afternoon (Sunday) at the baby shower of a very close friend. Carol, her daughter Lori, my daughter Melanie, and I all rode together. It was a lovely, well-attended shower with great food. Heather received many nice gifts and it was fun chatting and catching up with people I hadn't seen in quite some time.

During the course of the afternoon, I found out that I am on another prayer list at another church of another old friend. I received many hugs, and "You'll do just great" remarks. Thank goodness I am resting in the arms of the *One* who is my strength and upholds me in love. Because even though everyone thinks I am strong, my strength comes from above.

Well, I know I will need my strength for tomorrow, so I am going back to bed and try to rest. Surgery seemed so far away for a while, and now it is right before me.

Holy cow! The hospital called and gave me one surgery time, and then I received a call from Dr. Gold's office saying that in order to eliminate me having to wait until 5:30 p.m. tomorrow, my surgery has been changed to Friday, the 18 at 11:30 a.m.

Evidently the hospital did not have confirmation from Dr. Gold, only Dr. Pummill when the original time and date was set. Dr. Gold's receptionist did not seem happy, but early Friday is better with me. So now it's the old waiting game again.

I will journal more, either at the end of this week or while I am in for my hospital stay.

It is Wednesday, September 16, hump day. I actually slept pretty well last night. I only woke up two times, and I feel pretty rested. So, I have decided to continue in a positive vein. I have been trying to mop the bathroom floors, as well as the kitchen floor, so that my guys won't have to do much in that area. Today, I have decided to dust all the furniture in the bedrooms and in the living/dining areas. I am trying to keep the house as clean and neat as possible before my surgery Friday.

While I'm still able to, I went to the grocery store and stocked up on food for my guys and myself. I did the dishes and then I decided to make chocolate/peanut butter no-bake cookies for my husband, Mike, and my son, Chad. I also made Chad's favorite macaroni salad.

Then I cleaned out the dryer vent and wiped out the dryer tub with a damp cloth. With all that finished, I did two loads of laundry, and now I think I'll go outside and mow in the back one more time, while I can still enjoy this beautiful weather as well as be productive. Mowing is one of my favorite things to do, plus the lawn always looks so nice after it is mowed. The dogs seem to enjoy the shorter grass, too.

It really helps to keep my mind and myself busy, and then I don't feel so stressed.

I received another phone call from Deanna at Community Bible Church to check on me and find out the final details about the date and time of my surgery so that I may continue to be placed on their prayer list. It is really nice to have so many people supporting me with their love, concern, and prayers. I am truly blessed to have so many nice friends and loved ones behind me.

Just received a phone call from Vicki DeFloria, my nurse advocate from Blue Cross Blue Shield of Michigan (BCBS). Because of my diabetes, they have been contacting me to see how I am doing, as far as control. And when they found out about my breast cancer, my name was given to Vicki.

She has called me several times now to ask if I have any questions about the surgery, what I am to expect after, and just to lend me support. I sure do have a lot of people that are concerned about me. It really makes me feel special, even though I know there are many others, besides myself that have gone through this.

Anyway, it was really nice to hear from Vicki, and she said she would be calling the hospital to check up on me and then call me about a week after I come home.

Cleaning and dusting is done. Dishes are done. At dinner Tuesday night, Mike informed me that he would like to take me out to dinner when he comes home from work today (Wednesday). He said, "Your choice. Wherever you would like to go." What a treat! Now I guess I will just relax and watch a little television.

Well, just one more day home and then I will need to rise early on Friday, take a shower, and head to Dr. Pummill's office by 8:00 a.m. She will get me all marked up for surgery, and then I will cross Holly Road and enter the hospital where I will be checked into the surgery floor and preparations will begin for my big day.

Dinner out with Mike was great. We had a wonderful fish dinner and we enjoyed the beautiful weather, but mostly, we enjoyed just being with each other. We then came home and sat outside by the fire next to our decorative burner and enjoyed the quiet, the warm glow of the fire, and each other's company. Eventually I was out there by myself enjoying the solitude.

Today is Thursday, September 17 and I am trying to prepare for my early morning wake-up call and then the surgery that awaits me tomorrow.

My brother-in-law, whom I don't usually hear from, called this morning because he thought my surgery had already taken place on Tuesday. His first words to me were, "Oh, you're home already?"

I replied that the surgery had been postponed until Friday. He then asked me if I had gotten a second opinion. I told David that I had enough tests, needle biopsies, MRI's and genetic testing to help me make this decision, and that I knew this was something that had to be done. I also told him that because I am in the 50% and higher range for ovarian cancer that would have to be taken care of down the road.

Dave is still on the phone with Mike, giving him support and finding out how he is coping with all of this. It was really nice and unexpected that David called.

*Thank you Lord for the kindness of people.*

Well, it is back to finishing my laundry this morning and getting my clothes laid out for Friday morning. I will journal more, but I am not sure how many days will pass before I feel up to writing again.

It is now Thursday afternoon, around 1:20 p.m. I just spoke to Dr. Gold about a half hour ago. She called to thank me for an e-mail I sent her telling her how much I appreciate her, her sense of humor, her knowledge, and her kindness. After a little small talk, I asked her if the results were in from the final MRI needle biopsy I had last Friday, and she said, "Yes." They had come in late last night and the three satellite tumors were also malignant. She said, "Now we have all the facts and we know that we are making the right decision."

She told me she would see me in the morning and to get some rest. I asked her about when I could wash my hair and shower. I'm such a girly girl that I am used to showering and washing my hair every day. Dr. Gold said it would be one to two weeks. Since I will have drains in each breast, they don't really want me to get them wet and possibly cause an infection. Maybe I'll at least be able to use a dry shampoo and sponge bathe.

Another nice surprise, Harry, one of our neighbors came into the garage while Mike and I were in there talking. He asked how we were doing and offered to help in any way we needed. Then he gave me a big hug and told me that he and Joan (his wife) would be thinking of me tomorrow and that I would be fine. See what I mean about kindness and support from so many? I wish words could express fully how much it means to me.

So once again, I say, *Thank you Lord for these little blessings you keep bestowing on me. They help to uplift and strengthen me.*

And so, it is relax for the rest of the afternoon. Early to bed, early to rise, and then on to surgery.

Tonight was full of phone calls: Nancy, my sister-in-law Sheila from Tennessee, my sister-in-law Juanita from Drummond Island, my mother- and father-in-law, and the hospital giving me final instructions on arrival time and where to go to check in.

A really nice surprise was when three of my neighbors and their children stopped by with a lovely yellow mum in a wrought iron holder that reads, "Welcome," a card, and all their best wishes for a successful surgery and a speedy recovery, along with several hugs.

My son Chad just came home with a gift bag from the young lady he's been seeing. Inside was a lovely candle, an exfoliating sponge, heat-warming booties that soothe and soften your tootsies, and a manicure kit. All to pamper me after surgery.

Not such a bad way to end the day before surgery, ha! And with that I say, "Good night." Six o'clock in the morning comes all too soon.

It is 6:00 a.m. Friday morning, September 18, 2009. No breakfast — yuk. I took my pills, showered with anti-bacterial soap as directed by the hospital, and got dressed. No makeup or deodorant allowed, but I did manage a few squirts of cologne.

What can I say? I'm a girly girl.

I took the dogs out, than fed them their treats and their breakfast. Wrote one thank you card to MJ for her lovely and unexpected pampering gift. Waiting for Mike to finish getting ready and I'M OFF TO THE RACES!

It's 8:00 a.m. and I've arrived at Dr. Pummill's office to get marked for surgery and then I go directly across the street to the hospital entrance. Before I checked in, I stopped at Dr. Gold's office because I have a small gift to drop off to her first.

I am now on the second floor in the pre-op area and was asked to be seated and wait until my name is called. That didn't take very long, only about 15 minutes. It seems there a lot of people getting ready for surgeries today. I am taken to the prep area (pre-op) where I must change into one of their beautiful gowns, and then my IV was started. Next up: nuclear medicine. There I will have dye injected into each breast to locate the duct trail. The left breast is still so swollen and sore that the shot brought tears to my eyes.

Now I am taken back to pre-op where my friends Joyce and John Hovis are waiting with Mike. They are old friends from First Baptist Church of Pontiac, where Mike and I were married 40 years ago. They prayed with me and told me I would be just fine. That is the last thing I remember. Mike said they gave me a sedative, and it must have been a strong one, because I don't even remember saying goodbye to Mike or being wheeled into the surgery area.

I didn't get to see her before surgery, but my friend Nancy also came to the hospital, so she was able to talk with Mike, Joyce, and John.

The actual surgery lasted seven hours, and I guess I was in the recovery room about an hour before I was brought into my private room (not too shabby, huh?). It was really restful being in a room by myself though, so I am very thankful it was available to me.

The first thing I remember, after being in my room for a while, was seeing the faces of my husband, my son, and my dad. I remember they gave me some ice chips because my mouth was so dry, but they didn't stay down for very long. I think I vomited three times. My guys said I was really out of it.

I remember hurting really bad along the sides of each breast area and under my left arm. I couldn't move my arms hardly at all. They had me on morphine, and I remember the pain subsiding almost within minutes of receiving the morphine.

I slept really well that first night until about 4:30 a.m. I remember trying to eat a graham cracker, and it didn't stay down either, so I was given more nausea medication and fell back to sleep until 7:30 a.m. At that time I ate a saltine cracker and drank some water.

Thankfully, this time everything stayed down.

Breakfast came at 8:30 a.m. and the nurse's aide fed me some French toast and a little Special K cereal. I didn't feel like eating too much, but at least it stayed down, so that was great.

Then it was time for a glucose check and more pain medication so that I could rest comfortably again. Dr. Pummill came in to check my drains and my wounds. She was really pleased with the way I looked and my progress. She told me she would come in again on Sunday morning.

Later on Saturday afternoon, my friend Nancy Grimmer came to visit me for awhile. Bless her heart. She was there during the surgery on Friday, and I didn't even know it. She asked to see my wounds, so the nurse showed her. She told Mike if he needed any help not to hesitate to call upon her.

Had more company this afternoon: my dad, my daughter Melanie, Chad, and then my family physician, Dr. Kia arrived. What a nice day of surprise visits.

Each day I am more comfortable and able to walk to the bathroom and move my arms a little bit more.

I had some real excitement Saturday night, when everyone was visiting me. The nurse was draining my Jackson-Pratt (JP) drains*, while Chad sat at the end of the bed in a chair. We were talking about the color of the drainage and all of a sudden the nerve in the neck that sends messages to the brain, told my son's body to go into shock and he passed out in the chair. My husband hurried over to him so that he wouldn't hit the floor, and Melanie came over immediately to help also. Chad turned green and his heart rate dropped to 39.

The nurse wanted him to go the emergency room, but Chad refused. Melanie and Mike put their arms under his armpits and helped him to lie down on the sofa. He came around and said he felt better. He was given some juice and Mike went down to the food court in the hospital and brought him up some warm cookies. I guess all the stress of seeing me like I was, and seeing the blood being poured and measured out really got to him.

* A surgical drainage device used to pull excess fluid from the body by constant suction.

They left at 9:30 p.m., so I decided to turn out my lights and rest also. Boy. Chad sure scared me.

It is now Sunday morning, September 20, 2009, and I am awake and writing in my journal. It is only 5:20 a.m., but I feel rested. I need to go to the bathroom and I feel like eating another saltine, as I am a little hungry.

I laid back down and it is now 7:00 a.m., and I am cleaning out my JP drains myself. I also cleaned my face and put on some moisturizer. Slowly, but surely I am feeling a little better. I'm going to brush my teeth and then sit up in the chair and wait for breakfast. Then I think I'll take a little walk around the hall.

Dr. Pummill just arrived to check me again, and she is releasing me to go home. All I have to do now is get one final antibiotic in my IV, sign some release papers, get dressed, and then it's home, "James." The best news of all is that I do not need radiation or chemo!

My first full day home — Monday, September 21, 2009. I awoke at 7:00 a.m., came downstairs and ate some Wheaties and a piece of wheat toast. Took all my meds (I was a little nauseated). I also needed to take some MiraLAX, as I haven't experienced a bowel movement since Thursday (they told me the one med I am taking can cause that).

Mike helped me take a shower and wash my head. That was the most refreshing shower. It felt wonderful. I saw myself for the first time since surgery. I guess I don't look too bad from what Dr. Pummill said, but at least the cancer is gone.

I decided to write a little more in my journal before I take a little nap. I have gotten several phone calls during the day from people and family checking up on me: Dr. Pummill's office, Barb Wiser, my mother-in-law, Joyce Hovis, Nancy Grimmer, and my next-door neighbors. It's really nice to know people really care and are so supportive.

I think our dogs must have missed me, too, because they haven't left my side since I came home yesterday. Duke is right by my feet on the floor next to my chair. Gizzmo has his head laying on my leg on the La-Z-Boy next to me, and Raven is beside me. Charlie, well Charlie is old and just kind of does his own thing, but he did manage a kiss on the hand.

Mike just went to the grocery store to get me some soups and fruit for later. I have a great husband. He is such a big help to me.

Dr. Gold's office made an appointment for me this Thursday to remove the JP drains, and Dr. Pummill's office made a follow-up appointment for me this coming Monday.

I am still feeling a little nauseated, so I am trying to eat little meals, but eating more frequently. All in all, I guess my first full day at home hasn't been too bad. I just ate some vegetable soup with crackers and drank half a can of my diet pop. Time for more pain pills and I will probably have to lay down again, as the pills make me loopy. More tomorrow.

It is my second full day home, Tuesday, September 22, and I am feeling better today than I did before. Yesterday, it seemed every time I took a Vicodin I got really nauseous and had to lay down, even though I am only taking half a pill. Today, I think I will go without the meds and see how I do. Can't take being sick to my stomach.

Also, I finally had a bowel movement. It has been five days since I went, so it is no wonder my stomach felt a little funny. Anyway, I have been eating a little better today and was able to take a shower again this morning with Mike's help.

I have emptied my JP drains twice already today and noticed that the color is changing to a light pink now, so that is a really good sign also.

Three more cards came today and several more phone calls of people checking up on me and wishing me a speedy recovery. This is probably my best day so far, and hopefully, they will continue to get better and better each day.

On Wednesday, I took my first shower by myself (including washing and drying my hair) and got completely dressed on my own this morning. It feels good to have clothes on instead of a nightgown all day, which makes me feel a little more human. According to the doctors, I am doing quite well.

Mike helped me make pancakes for breakfast, and I did the morning dishes. Now I am doing a load of wash, but I didn't carry the laundry basket; I'm only allowed to put the clothes in the washing machine and in the dryer. Mike and Chad always help me unload the dryer and fold the clothes. Now, I think I will sit back and relax on the computer for a while. So far, so good this morning.

Today is Thursday, September 24, 2009, and I just left Dr. Gold's office, where I was hoping to have the JP drains removed; no luck. There is still enough drainage coming from each side that to remove the drains would put me at risk for infection and fluid buildup in the wounds themselves. I guess I can wait four more days until I see the plastic surgeon, to have them taken out. It is just a little difficult to sleep when I happen to roll over on them because they pull a little, and they are a little trouble when I shower.

I feel like it was a three steps forward and then two steps back kind of a day. I was told that in the right breast not only was there a 1.5-centimeter mass behind the nipple, but there was a small infiltrating tumor, as there were three of the same in the left breast.

All the breast tissue has been removed, so they are all gone, but because of the size of the tumor in the left breast (2 centimeters) an automatic Oncotype DX® breast recurrence test is being done in California. It will determine if I am at risk between 0 – 100 for reoccurrence within ten years. If my results come back in the low-risk range, then I only need to take the estrogen-blocking drug and I am all set. If my results come back in the intermediate range, there is a possibility of chemo as well as the estrogen-blocking drug. And if my results come back in the high-risk range, then chemo is imminent.

*Please Lord. Let me be selfish. Let this test come back in the low-risk range. I just want to be able to heal now without the loss of my hair and feeling totally tired with no energy for a period of 14 weeks.*

Now it is a waiting game again for two to three weeks until the report comes back from California. My surgeon has no real say in the treatment. This test is totally dependent upon the oncologist's report and findings.

Trying to stay positive is a little difficult today, but with God's help, "This too shall pass." Each cancer is different in its cell construction, which is why this test is done. It has nothing to do with the genetic testing, it has to do with the actual construction of the cancer cells that are in the biopsy samples.

It is Saturday morning, September 26, and I am feeling a little better about the Oncotype DX testing that is being done on my breast tissue, right at this moment in California. I went to their website to gain more information and view the video they have that further explains the process.

I now realize that I am very lucky to be living in a day and age where this state-of-the-art, accurate, and reliable genes tumor testing is readily available. California is the only state where this remarkable facility is located.

It is another diagnostic tool for the surgeon and patient to use in helping to decide on the best course of treatment after surgery. It allows both to be aware of the possibility of recurrence within a ten-year span, and it also helps to make chemo available to those who need it, as well as those who will not benefit from chemo.

The Oncotype DX was tested in a large clinical trial study of women with stage I or II nodes, negative, estrogen receptor positive (ER+) breast cancer. The trial recurrence score accurately predicts the likelihood of breast cancer recurrence.

You are scored on a range from 0 – 100 in three categories: low risk, intermediate risk, and high risk for recurrence. If you are in the low-risk area usually an estrogen-blocking medication is prescribed and no chemo is necessary.

If you progress to a low/intermediate risk area, the same is usually prescribed. However, if you enter the intermediate/high or high-risk area, then chemo is usually added to the medication therapy so that the patient can feel comfortable that there will be no recurrence in the ten-year time span.

Even though chemo was not a word I wanted to hear five days after my surgery, I now realize how important this test is in determining the course of my future treatment. However, I am praying in a selfish way, that my results come back in the low-risk area. I am starting to feel better each day, and I do not relish the idea of being totally fatigued *and* losing my hair.

It was a beautiful fall weekend with lots of sunshine and crisp air. Mike and I enjoyed a Saturday together, going to a harvest day at a local nursery. We picked up some beautiful amber-colored mums and some cornstalks for the front porch. It is wonderful to be able to do the little things again that make life so fulfilling and exciting. I love to decorate my porch for the holidays and fall is one of my favorite times.

Today is Monday, September 28, 2009, and I am making another trek to the plastic surgeon's office. I am hoping to have these JP drains removed so that the area around it can fully heal and I will be able to take a shower without having to put the drains in a towel around my neck, and without having to fight with them while I am trying to dress. It will also be wonderful to be able to turn a little in bed without laying on the drain bottles or the lines surrounding them.

I also have some questions for Dr. Pummill about how I am progressing in the healing category, and if I will be able to receive my flu shot soon. I surely don't want to get the flu on top of all that has transpired in my body.

My spirit feels strong this beautiful, but chilly morning, and I have hope for healing and for the future. I feel very blessed again to have such a great team of doctors, surgeons, and plastic surgeons working with me and as advocates for me.

YAAAAAAAHHHHHHHOOOOOOOOO!

The JP drains are out! I felt a little pinch when the stitches were cut and the drain line was pulled, but I am so thankful to have them out. Now I can move a little freer, and I feel like the umbilical cord to my breast cancer surgery has been cut. I should be able to sleep a little better, and shower a little easier, too.

Now I have to apply my antibiotic cream to both the surgical areas and the drain holes twice a day to prevent any infection until the holes seal themselves up.

77

When I was in the procedure room, the technician told me I looked great, and I began to cry. I know I will never look the same way again, but they say I am right where I should be, as far as the healing process goes. And that I have a positive attitude, and the shape of the skin under the tissue expanders looks really good.

Dr. Pummill told me not to worry about the tears — they are perfectly normal after a surgery of this magnitude. She told me she would see me again next Monday morning, October 5, 2009.

Wow. October all ready.

Anyway, I am home now and just had lunch with my husband.

*Thank you Lord for a supportive, caring, and loving husband, who has been traveling on this journey, right by my side.*
*I am so blessed.*

It's Wednesday, September 30 ,2009, and I have a real case of the doldrums today. Not sure why. I know it has only been one week and five days since my surgery. As I see my wounds each morning and evening, I get teary eyed. It feels almost like I am mourning the loss of what I had.

I know that beauty comes from within, and I am still the same person I was before inside, but I look so totally different on the outside. I also know this is not permanent, as far as the cosmetics are concerned, but the scars will be around for quite a long time, if not forever.

*Lord, give me the patience and strength I need as I recover. Help me to take it one minute, one hour, one day, one week, and one month at a time.*

After I applied the antibiotic ointment to my wounds, my husband just gave me a big hug and told me I was beautiful. He said, "I have you, and you have your life. Don't worry about what others say or think. You still have me."

I am so blessed, Lord. Thank you for my better half and his love and support through this whole journey. He just uplifted me with his sweet words.

It is Saturday, October 3, 2009, and Mike and I have decided to go to the cider mill today, even though it is a dreary day. When we arrived inside the mill, the smell of fresh donuts permeated the air. We decided to buy a dozen sugared donuts and a half-gallon of cold cider. Both items hit the spot; the donuts were still warm and melted in our mouths, and the cold cider washed them down nicely.

We then decided to drive through Milford to enjoy the rest of the afternoon. As we did, the sun finally came out. It seems as though all we did was eat on Saturday, because we decided to stop at the Big Boy Restaurant for Slim Jim sandwiches before heading home.

Even after over 40 years of marriage, we still enjoy each other's company. Weekends for us are precious.

The weekend flew by, and it is now Monday, October 5, 2009, and I just arrived back home from Dr. Pummill's office. She assured me that I am healing wonderfully and that I can begin to increase my activity level. I just need to listen to my body, and if I hurt or grow extremely tired, I am to stop and rest.

I was also told that I could now start driving again and that when I return to her office next Monday, October 12, the stretching process will begin. She will increase the amount of saline in the temporary implants.

The following Thursday, October 15, I returned to see Dr. Gold. Hopefully, the results from the Oncotype DX test will be back, and I will find out whether or not chemo is required for the healing process. You already know what I'm wishing for — no chemo!

Anyway, it is onward and upward with my journey.

It's another full weekend (Mike's birthday) and we're going to enjoy being out in the crisp fall air at a car show in Armada, Michigan. Just my guys and me: my dad, my son, and my husband spending the day together.

Tomorrow morning, I return to Dr. Pummill's office where she will be injecting more saline solution into each of the tissue expanders in both breasts. The procedure is a slow one, but the only way to stretch the skin gradually to make room for the permanent implants. I think the whole process will take three to four months, depending on how I progress and how I tolerate the pain.

The whole procedure only took about ten minutes. A small needle was injected into the port of the tissue expanders, and more saline was injected into each side. I experienced some minor discomfort, but it wasn't too bad. Dr. Pummill told me I would probably be sore tonight, to the point where I might need to take a pain pill. I am a little sore at the moment, so I am trying not to use my arms any more than I absolutely need to.

Another appointment was made for next Monday morning, the 19, where the same procedure will be repeated once again. I asked about how many times I would need to return, and Dr. Pummill told me about four. It really all depends on how I am progressing size wise. I told her I didn't want to look like Dolly Parton, and she just laughed.

On Thursday, October 15, I will return to Dr. Gold's office for the Oncotype DX test results.

Pain.

PAIN.

PPPAAAIIINNN!

It is Wednesday morning about 4:00 a.m., and I woke with a throbbing pain in both sides of my chest. It hurt so bad that I had to get up from the La-Z-Boy where I was trying to sleep, and eat something so that I could take a pain pill. It hurts even more to raise my arms, and the pain extends around to my back.

I called the doctor's office later in the morning to ask if this was normal. Unfortunately, it is. They suggested I use ice packs and pain pills during the day, so that is the regime that I am on today. It does seem to help, but I guess I was surprised at the amount of pain I had earlier. It almost feels as bad as it did the day after I had surgery.

Hopefully, it will decrease with each passing day. I am wondering if I will experience this each time I have to go in for more saline injections into the temporary tissue spacers. I can't imagine anyone going through breast implants just for the fun of it, because it isn't a walk in the park.

I will continue to use the ice packs today, and I just took another half of a pain pill with my dinner. Let's hope that tomorrow is better.

It is Thursday, October 15, 2009, and I attended my first breast cancer fundraising event today. Hank Graff, the automobile dealership in Davison, Michigan was the sponsor. For every $10.00 charged to drive a new vehicle, they matched the dollar amount. I was able to drive a brand-new Camaro. Holy cow! That car has get-up-and-go, and Mike and I got up and went!

I met some really nice cancer survivors there. One lady is a three-time cancer survivor who will be on chemo the rest of her life. Another lady I met had a daughter-in-law that had a double mastectomy, and she also underwent reconstructive surgery.

The one lady in the booth gave me a big hug, and thanked me for attending, even though I am only three weeks out of surgery. She also gave me a breast cancer pink ribbon/angel pendant to wear.

I called Dr. Pummill's office today to reschedule my Monday appointment. I told them I was just too sore to undergo another round of saline injections right now. They told me there was no problem in delaying this procedure for another week. Hopefully the next appointment will not leave me quite as sore as this first visit did.

I will continue to use my ice packs and take my pain pills for the next couple of days until I am not quite so uncomfortable.

It has been several days since I have felt like journaling. It seems my mental attitude has been under attack.

At the end of last week (October 16) I received a phone call from Oncotype DX in California where my cancer tissue is being tested. Evidently my insurance will pay for testing on the one breast, but since I had cancer in both sides, my surgeon wants to get the other breast tissue tested, also. Onco assured me that they will submit more information to BCBS in order for this to be taken care of, but there is still a possibility that it won't be paid for. If that is the case, I will need to send Onco my W2 information. If our income is less than $72,000 for the entire year, then I am prequalified, and Onco will write-off the added expense.

At the same time, Mike received two more bills from Dr. Young's (his physician) office for his physical, and from Dr. Kia (my doctor) for my remaining balance on my physical. It seems the stress of all these bills has put us both on edge and makes us snap at each other. I know the cancer was not my fault, but because of my illness, I feel like all these added bills have put a strain on our lives.

Also, last week was a really uncomfortable one for me. Tuesday morning after meeting with Dr. Pummill on Monday for the saline injections into the tissue expanders, I woke up with a throbbing pain, particularly in my left breast. It took me all of that same week to start feeling more comfortable.

Because of that discomfort, I had a night where I found it hard to sleep, so I had to take another pain pill and I also had a crying spell. I keep thinking to myself that I wish the discomfort was over, and that the permanent implants were already in place. Maybe this sounds a little selfish (after all, it's only been a month after my surgery) but I really don't do well with pain and these temporary tissue expanders are hard.

It feels, at times, like my arms are right up against them and that I don't have a lot of ability to lift my arms, or even place my arms comfortably against the sides of my chest.

On a positive note, I am feeling more comfortable now, and I will be going to see Dr. Pummill next Monday where I will have a chance to address these issues with her.

It has been one month and a week since I had my surgery, and it is really wonderful to know that people are still concerned about the progress I am making in my recovery stage. I am still getting phone calls and cards from friends and relatives, wishing me well and inquiring as to how I am doing.

Tomorrow morning, October 26, 2009, I need to be in Dr. Pummill's office at 8:15 a.m. for my second round of saline injections into the tissue spacers. I need to ask her questions about the discomfort I have experienced to know whether or not it's normal.

I also want to ask her how far out she feels the next surgery will be to replace the temporary tissue expanders with the permanent silicone implants. Maybe I'll have them by Christmas. We'll see.

It hardly seems possible, but Halloween is next weekend, and then we look forward to Thanksgiving and then, in just two months, Christmas will be upon us.

I feel like I am making good progress, even though there has been a lot of discomfort with these tissue expanders. Hopefully, this next time it will be somewhat less painful for me. Other than that, I feel really good and I am actually starting to have a little shape on top again. That feels and looks great, even though I still will have some scaring. I am sure in time that will dissipate, too.

Until tomorrow's appointment with the plastic surgeon, I will sign off for now.

It's Monday, October 26, 2009 and I just returned from Dr. Pummill's office where I had my second saline injections into the tissue spacers. This time, I took an extra-strength Tylenol before I went into her office in hopes of alleviating some of the discomfort I experienced two weeks ago.

While there, I had the opportunity to ask Dr. Pummill about all the discomfort that I experienced, and she explained that when the nerve endings start to regenerate, that everything becomes super sensitive, and that is why I am so uncomfortable. I asked her also how many more visits I would need before we took out the temporary tissue spacers and replace them with the permanent silicone implants. She told me four more visits. I then asked her for a target date for the permanent implants, and she told me December 30, 2009. I should have new boobs for the New Year. Yahoo!

After my appointment with Dr. Pummill, I stopped across the street to see my family physician, Dr. Kia. I wanted to show her my "bumps," and also to say hello. She was not in the office until 10:00 a.m., but I was able to say, "Hi" to her nurse, Judy. I talked to her for a few minutes and she asked to see my surgery results. She was impressed, and said I looked a lot better than many other patients she has seen.

That made me feel a lot better. Hopefully, when I go to see Dr. Kia in January, I will be able to show them how good my new "boobs" look. Anyway, so much for writing today. I think I am going to go downstairs and sit in the La-Z-Boy with a pillow under my arms. That seems to help to take some of the pressure off me.

It has been four days since I had my second saline injections into the tissue spacers. I have not been quite as uncomfortable this time as I was with the first session. I know that the tissue expanders are not meant for comfort, they are meant to expand the tissue to get ready for the permanent silicone implants.

The doctor has given me a prescription for a numbing cream containing Lidocaine and Prilocaine. It is a topical cream that is meant to numb the area where the needle is inserted. She feels that this might help with the discomfort also. I need to apply the cream one hour before going to the doctor.

I only have four more sessions with the injections and then I can look forward to getting the permanent implants on December 30, 2009. My only concern now is that when I see my surgeon, Dr. Gold on November 4, I will find out whether or not I need chemo. If I do need chemo, I wonder if it will affect the date of my scheduled surgery. I guess that is another one of those questions that I need to direct to Dr. Gold. I am still hoping that the test results show that I am in the low recurrence range and that I will only need to take the estrogen-blocking medication for five years.

One positive is that I am able to increase my activities. I find that if I get too uncomfortable, I just stop what I am doing, and then pick up that activity later. I went shopping by myself the other day for a few Christmas gifts. I found that after an hour I started to hurt, so I finished up and came home.

I am still getting cards, phone calls, and encouragement from friends and loved ones. Wish they knew how much it means to be remembered. Thank you all.

Today, November 2, 2009, I visited Dr. Pummill again for the third saline injection. The numbing cream she prescribed for me actually helped take the edge off the area where she needed to insert the needle. I am really sore right now though. It feels like my skin can't stretch anymore, but Dr. Pummill said there is still room for more cc's.

I was supposed to go back to Dr. Gold's office this Wednesday, but Mike's uncle Dick passed away this past Sunday morning, and the funeral is scheduled for Wednesday at 1:00 p.m. So I called Dr. Gold's office today and rescheduled my appointment for Thursday, November 5 at 2:30 p.m.

At this appointment, I am supposed to find out the results of the cancer tissue tests, and the likelihood of the cancer returning within the next ten years.

I am still hoping and praying that my level of recurrence is in the low area so that I will just need to take the estrogen-blocking medication.

Today I found out from Dr. Pummill that if it is necessary that I need chemo treatments, my second surgery to put the silicone implants in will have to be delayed. Another reason to hope that it comes back in the low range, right? Anyway, I have a funeral to focus on right now, so Thursday's appointment will have to be put on the back burner for now. More to write about later.

It is Thursday, November 5, 2009, and I just left Dr. Gold's office with some good news and some great news. The good news is that the left breast cancer tissue results showed that the recurrence rate is 27, which is in the moderate range. The great news is that the right breast cancer tissue results came back and showed that my recurrence rate is 15, which is in the low range.

She explained to me that I need to go see an oncologist so that the estrogen-blocking medication can be prescribed. It will be necessary for me to stay on this medication for a five-year period, and I will need to be monitored to make sure that I am doing well on the medication.

The oncologist may encourage me to take chemo because of the moderate level report on the left breast, but I feel that since both breasts were removed, the lymph nodes were all clear, and the low-to-moderate cancer tissue reports all make me feel that I can go on with the healing process now. I will be getting two more saline injections into the tissue spacers, and then my second surgery is still scheduled for December 30, 2009.

I will have new boobs for the New Year. Hooray!!

Yesterday was my last visit to the plastic surgeon's office until December 21, 2009. That is the pre-op appointment for my implant surgery, which is scheduled for December 30.

I wish I could say that the appointment went well, but I actually got physically ill and vomited when the saline was injected. I am really quite uncomfortable today, and I am hoping that within the next day or two, I will start feeling human again.

I was supposed to go to the oncologist's office tomorrow, but I rescheduled the appointment for next week because of my discomfort level. They were very kind on the phone and understood my dilemma. I feel like every time I journal lately it is to complain about my pain, but I am trying to be honest, and I guess my discomfort level needs to be put in here also.

Because of my pain, I am not able to continue my regular activities, and I think that is what bothers me the most. I take my shower every morning, brush my teeth, dress myself (sometimes with help), and then I return to the La-Z-Boy chair where I take my pain meds and then just sit and relax.

This journey is not over yet, but at least I can see the light at the end of the tunnel, and I *know* that the final results will be worth it.

I haven't written in my journal for the last few days because there isn't much happening at this point of my journey. I had my last saline injections last week with a lot of discomfort, but things are getting better in the pain department. I still find that I am resting better at night if I take a pain pill before I retire. It helps to relax me and I can actually almost sleep throughout the night. I still need to sleep in the La-Z-Boy, but I am getting used to that also.

On Friday, November 20, I have an appointment with Dr. Rizwan Danish, the oncologist, at which time I will be receiving my prescription for the estrogen-blocking medication. I already know that I will need to stay on the medication for a five-year period. I am hoping that I do not have any, or at least, very few reactions (such as hot flashes) with this medication.

People are still contacting me and asking about my progress. It is very uplifting to still be getting cards and phone calls, and know that people are supporting me. I am feeling much better and getting more use to these tissue expanders, although my breasts feel like rocks right now, and I feel like my skin can't stretch any further. At least I know it won't be much longer before they come out and the permanent silicone implants are in place.

Yesterday, I was faced with the fact life is short and that we need to make each day count. I placed a grave blanket on my mother's grave for the winter season. My husband and I walked around in the area where his uncle Irwin is supposed to be located. We didn't find his grave, but there were several other headstones we came across that were those of teenagers.

On one of the graves, for a beautiful young lady, there was a lovely poem on her headstone that actually brought tears to my eyes, and an ache in my heart for the parents left behind to mourn.

I am thankful that my cancer has been taken care of, and that I am still here to enjoy the holidays and the little things that others may take for granted.

Today is November 18, 2009. It is my 62$^{nd}$ birthday — a day I truly didn't know for sure if I would be celebrating a few months ago. When you are initially diagnosed with cancer, the first thing you think is that you are not going to be around for long. Your second reaction is a feeling of numbness, and the third reaction (at least in my case) was I *am* going to fight this thing!

I am so thankful to all my doctors: Dr. Manisha Kia (primary care physician), Dr. Linsey Gold (cancer surgeon), and Dr. Kimberly Pummill (plastic surgeon).

All of these talented, smart doctors make up my support team, and I thank them all from the bottom of my heart that I have this day and many others
to celebrate another year of life with my family.

Now I am off to make a birthday cake for myself, and to share it with Mike, Melanie, my grandchildren, Chad, and my father.

HAPPY BIRTHDAY TO ME:
CELEBRATE LIFE!

My appointment with Dr. Danish was today. He has a sense of humor, which I enjoyed. His first sentence to me was, "Is this your father?"

I replied, "No. It's my husband!"

He then said to my husband, "Oh, you've got a young one."

Perhaps that was his way of breaking the ice with Mike and I. I guess I look a little younger than Mike.

And what woman doesn't love being told she looks younger?

He looked over all my pathology reports, the reports from the Oncotype DX testing, and asked me about the genetic testing that I had done. I was also asked about my family history regarding the breast cancer, and I told him I was the first in my family to experience it.

He left the room for a few minutes, and then returned with a sheet of paper that he asked Mike and I both to look at while he went over it with us. It showed the percentage of me being alive in ten years without any additional therapy. The result was 88.0 percent. The report also showed the benefit of hormonal therapy, which was only 0.9 percent.

The percentage of me dying with cancer was 2.9 percent.

And if you deduct the 0.9 percent with hormone therapy, which leaves a 2 percent chance left of dying with cancer. I felt that it was great news and that I really didn't need to take the estrogen-blocking medicine. However, Dr. Danish recommended that I take it for one month to see if I have any adverse reactions to it. He told me if I did that I could discontinue taking it.

I will need to see him again in one month (December 18) to see how I am doing on the medication. He also asked me to get a bone-density test, and blood work to check my calcium level upon my next visit. It was also recommended that I start taking calcium and Vitamin D.

When I left his office and went back to the reception desk, I got a real shock when I was told that the fee for today's consultation was $229.00. Yesterday, I received two other doctor bills totaling $103.00 and then this large consultation fee today. I wish there were some way to help with these expenses.

It has been a little while since I have written in this journal, but there isn't a whole lot happening right now. I saw the oncologist a week ago, and I have been taking the estrogen-blocking medication, Arimidex, for a week now.

I have experienced some nausea and some constipation on this medication, so I am not sure how long I will actually take it. Dr. Danish told me it all depended on the quality of life. If I experienced any adverse reactions then I could discontinue taking it. He felt that it would not affect me very much if I did stop taking it.

In four weeks I will have my implant surgery, so right now I am focusing on the Christmas season with my family.

Yesterday, my husband, my son, and I went to cut down our Christmas tree. We also did a little Christmas shopping and today I decorated the tree. I love the holiday season with all the lights — everything looks so bright and festive. I also put up my nativity and my angels, and I was reminded of the guardian angels that have been with me throughout this journey.

I know God has me in his hands and that I am being protected.

I am also very thankful with the outcome I have experienced: I do not need chemotherapy, and it looks like I will not have to take the estrogen-blocking medication for long either. I am hoping that all goes as well during this second surgery. I am so very thankful for my health, and I will never take it for granted. Each day is precious, and I am very thankful that I am around and getting better each day to enjoy this wonderful time of the year and to reflect on the birth of the Saviour that loves me so very much.

I am so very thankful for my husband, Mike. He made a comment while I was preparing Thanksgiving dinner as to how much he would miss me; not just if I weren't here to prepare dinner, but each day of his life if I were gone. What a wonderful thing to say. How I am so very blessed by his presence in my life!

I have been on the telephone for several days, calling different organizations that were recommended to me by Vicki, my nurse advocate at Blue Cross Blue Shield of Michigan.

My husband and I are struggling to make all the necessary co-pays that have been coming to our house after my cancer surgery.

It seems that there really isn't much financial help unless you're a patient on chemotherapy treatments and you are taking medications on a continuous basis to fight your cancer. As a cancer survivor, I find this very frustrating and unfair. Everyone tells you to keep your chin up, stay positive, get well and heal, but they don't realize that all the financial stress takes a toll on the healing process.

I already cancelled the next appointment with my oncologist, Dr. Danish, because each time I go there is a $104.00 co-pay for office visits that my insurance program does not cover. The office manager for Dr. Danish told me about a program, available only through The Genesys Foundation, called "Reunion with a Cause," which offers one-time financial assistance to pay for heat, light, transportation, or a house payment.

However, the woman who was supposed to call me regarding this help never did. I wish there was some type of assistance for all the cancer patients that do not have to take chemotherapy or drug therapy during their healing process. I feel blessed that chemo is not needed in my case, but I am still very stressed over the bills that just keep coming.

After my second surgery on December 30, 2009, I know that I will be receiving more bills.

I think this is an area that our healthcare professionals and the insurance companies really need to look at closely when someone suffers from a catastrophic disease.

Cancer is a disease that no one wishes to get, and it really makes it hard on the rest of the family when there is this much stress because of finances.

It's been a couple of weeks since I have written in my journal, but things have slowed down quite a bit except for the hustle and bustle of the Christmas season; my favorite time of the year.

I am so thankful that I am well enough to shop for the ones I love, selecting just the right gift, and that I am well enough to enjoy the wonderful Christmas music that seems to permeate the air everywhere you go, and overall just enjoy this time of year with all my loved ones.

I am very thankful to say that I was able to receive a one-time monetary gift from "Reunion with a Cause." This will really help alleviate some of the stress my husband has been experiencing because of the co-pays from the doctor's office visits, medications, and co-pays from the surgery.

I would like to help next August with their fundraiser that takes place in Holly — to help other cancer patients with the same financial difficulties that we have experienced. I feel it is not just my duty to give back, but also a privilege to give back: I am doing well and getting ready for the next step in my journey. My permanent implant surgery is scheduled for December 30.

Maybe I can be some encouragement to someone experiencing this disease, because I feel I have been blessed with much support and love from many who know me. I will probably not journal too much until just before or possibly just after my second surgery. It will all depend on what I feel inspired to write and how well I will be able to type after the surgery. In the meantime, I wish everyone all the joy, love, and blessings during this blessed Christmas time. May God bless all of you going through this journey, as He has blessed me.

Today is Saturday, December 19, 2009. It hardly seems possible, but there are only six days 'till Christmas. I have been busy this morning walking Duke, my son's German Shepherd, shoveling a beautiful light snow from the deck, the driveway, and the sidewalk, and then I came into the house and baked some Christmas cookies. After that, I stripped off my bedding and did a load of wash.

It is really wonderful to be able to do even small things. After my double mastectomy, it was really hard for me to lift my arms for a long time. I am very thankful that I can do a lot of my regular tasks and activities again. However, in 11 days, I will be going in for my implant surgery, so I am sure that I will experience some soreness and loss of activity once again.

I received a phone call from plastic surgeon yesterday reminding me of my pre-op appointment with her Monday, December 21, 2009 at 9:15 a.m. Then, the oncologist's office called reminding me of my appointment the same day at noon.

I'm such a popular gal.

I am very much looking forward to Christmas and time with my family before I head off for another surgery. And I am praying all goes well.

The stockings are hung by the chimney with care, and the Christmas tree is adorned with ornaments and lights. All the shopping is done, the gifts are wrapped and the Christmas cookies are made, and yet I am in a blue mood. Why? I'm not sure. Maybe it is the culmination of all that I have been through, or maybe it is the fact that my father has been having a lot of pain in his hip and needs to go see the orthopedic surgeon. Or maybe it's the fact that both my children are out of work at this time, or maybe it is all of the above: Either way, I am not enjoying the holiday that I have always loved so much.

Instead, I find myself missing my mother, who passed away three years ago this January. Mom always made the holiday special with her singing of Christmas carols, her shopping for just the right gift for each person on her list, trimming her Christmas tree with such care and precision — placing each ornament in just the right spot.

All these memories are still precious, but the one who made them special is in the arms of Jesus this year.

I am hoping that by Friday, Christmas Day, I find myself joyful again in the company of loved ones I have not seen since last year, along with the excitement of opening gifts on Christmas morning after "Santa" has been here, and the realization that I am loved and protected by the *One* who was born on this special day and makes this holiday what it really is all about.
*Happy Birthday, Jesus.*

Today is Monday, December 21, 2009 and I had two doctor's appointments. The first appointment was with my plastic surgeon, Dr. Pummill. She went over the procedures for my breast implant surgery next Wednesday, December 30, 2209. She explained that I will have a little larger incision this time so that she can easily remove the tissue expanders on each side and position the permanent implants exactly where she wants them to be. She also told me that she doesn't anticipate any problems, and that I will do great again.

I asked about the discomfort level this time around, and she explained that I probably would not be as sore, if at all. That was music to my ears. I will not be able to have any activity as far as driving, lifting, or pushing for three weeks again, but I can handle that.

My second appointment today was with Dr. Danish. We discussed the side effects that occurred when I took the Arimidex, and we jointly decided that the effects were not worth taking the medication. However, Dr. Danish scheduled a vaginal ultrasound for me for next Tuesday, December 29, 2009 at 5:00 p.m.

He wants a clear picture of the condition of my ovaries at this time since I am BRCA2 positive. Then I will not need to see him again for six months, which takes me into June 2010.

While I was in the waiting room at Dr. Danish's office, a cancer volunteer was talking to each of us, and I overheard a conversation she was having with another lady, Lydia.

She had experienced breast cancer and she also had kidney cancer. Lydia had reconstructive surgery, so I struck up a conversation with her. Both she and her husband had nothing but glowing reports about my surgeon, Dr. Linsey Gold, and my plastic surgeon, Dr. Kimberly Pummill. They both said they are the best.

Lydia also told me she is in a breast cancer support group and offered me her phone number and address. She and her husband both told me that if I just wanted to, or needed to talk, to call — even if it was 2:00 a.m. I was really glad that I was able to meet and talk with them both today. It is nice to meet someone else who has already gone through everything that I have.

*Once again, thank you Lord for letting these people cross my path today. I know it was no mistake.*

It is December 28, 2009, and I am only two days away from my implant surgery.

Our family had a really nice, somewhat quiet Christmas. On Christmas Day, we had dinner at my sister-in-law's home, where we got to see many of the family members we hadn't seen since last year's event.

After dinner, Mike and I dropped my dad off at his home, and we spent the rest of the evening together quietly.

Tomorrow at 5:00 p.m. I am scheduled for a vaginal ultrasound at the Linden Road MRI building. This building is where I had my last computer-generated needle biopsy before my double mastectomy took place. I cannot have anything to eat for four hours prior to the procedure. Since I am BRCA2 positive, the oncologist wants to actually see the ovaries and the uterus to make sure that I don't have to worry about that surgery for a while. I guess it is better to be safe than sorry.

It is Tuesday, December 29, and I had the vaginal ultrasound. It was a snap, no pain at all. The lady that gave me the test asked if she could pray for me tonight, wishing me well tomorrow during surgery, and I told her, "Sure. You can never have too many prayers offered up."

When I got back home, my daughter Melanie called to tell me that she was coming to spend the night, so that she could go with me in the morning. That was a really nice surprise.

After that phone call, Vicki, the nurse advocate from the BCBS office, also called me to see how I was feeling about the procedure tomorrow.

I told her I was excited, but also a little nervous. She told me she would have another nurse, named Kathy, call me in the afternoon to check up on me after surgery. It is really nice to have all this support and good wishes.

I pray tomorrow goes really well.

On Wednesday, December 30, 2009, I will need to wake up at 5:00 a.m. so that I can shower and arrive at the outpatient building at 6:30 a.m. I will be prepped and then surgery is at 7:30 a.m.

I am very anxious to get the tissue expanders removed and replaced with the permanent implants, but at the same time I am nervous again. Dr. Pummill doesn't expect any problems, so I will trust her capable hands and once again keep faith in God. He hasn't failed me yet, and I know several people are still praying for me again during this procedure.

I'm not sure if I'll be able to journal right after surgery, because I really don't know how sore I will be, and once again my activities will be limited for three weeks.

Wednesday, December 30, I arrived at the surgery center at 6:30 a.m. to register, and was a little apprehensive because they couldn't find my files. Of course, they finally located it... in the wrong date pile. I was taken back to the pre-op area, and Melanie went back with me.

Dr. Pummill came in and I was able to introduce her to my daughter. Melanie asked how many cc's were going to be used in the implants. Dr. Pummill told her between 400-600 cc's of saline. Melanie said, "Go 700 cc's!" I told her I didn't want to look like Dolly Parton (I was assured I wouldn't).

My IV was started, which I'm always nervous about because of my small veins, but surprisingly, it wasn't as bad as I expected.

I was in surgery about an hour and 45 minutes, but I had to stay in recovery for three hours because I wasn't breathing hard enough through my nose and my respiration was dropping — and actually stopped for about 15 seconds.

The anesthesiologist thought I might have a slight problem with sleep apnea. Melanie thinks I just had a little too much anesthesia.

They sent me home with Keflex for infection, Phenergan for nausea, and Vicodin for pain. I vomited up a little water when I was in the post-op room and once again when I arrived home. All in all I feel really good, and I am not half as sore as I was with my first surgery.

I am very thankful the surgery is over, and I will be going to see Dr. Pummill tomorrow at 1:00 p.m. for my post-op visit. She will be removing some of the tape and actually looking at the incision area.

I can't wait to see my new set of boobs.

Thursday, December 31, 2009 and I just got home from Dr. Pummill's office. She said I looked great and is very pleased that I don't have any drainage and I am only slightly swollen. She told me there is a possibility I could still bruise a little bit, but overall she is really pleased with the results. And I can shower on Saturday.

I have another appointment next Thursday, January 7, 2010 where Dr. Pummill will give me an antibiotic cream to start applying to the wound areas. I should be pretty well healed in six weeks time.

At this time, I don't have much discomfort, and for that I am very thankful. I am just tolerating a little soreness in the breastbone area because that is where the skin was not stretched out quite as much as we would have liked.

Overall, I feel pretty normal again, and I feel I look more normal. Hopefully, I will look more like myself in my clothes this summer when I am out and about gardening in my yard.

Today is January 1, 2010.

It is a New Year and I feel like a new person. I am still a little bruised near my breastbone, and have a little soreness there. I've only had to take two pain pills since coming home, so I think that is pretty good.

I can't drive for three weeks, and I am really limited as to the activities I can do at this time, but I can still journal. That gives me something to keep my mind busy.

The computer printer broke here at home, so I am writing in longhand. I will have to figure out a way to type my current pages.

Last night my next-door neighbors Vicki and Jeff brought over a roasted chicken, chicken Alfredo pasta, and a pie. They have been extremely helpful, as they know I had my second surgery and they don't want me to cook. They also brought me a pink candle and a dozen pink shrub roses in a vase.

How nice to have such nice, caring neighbors.

It's been one week since my implant surgery. The wounds look great, and I have been really lucky that I have only had slight bruising. I really didn't experience pain this time as much as soreness. I have a 9:15 a.m. appointment with my plastic surgeon, Dr. Pummill tomorrow for another post surgery check-up.

With Mike back at work, I'm starting to get cabin fever. I'll really be glad when I get the OK to drive again. I love being able to get out and about a little bit.

I saw Dr. Pummill again on January 7, 2010 and she removed the steri-strips off both wounds. From now on I'll have to apply antibiotic cream two times a day on each breast, and then in 10 days I will return to Dr. Pummill's office. At the next visit, I will be getting scar cream to apply to help the scars disappear and become less apparent.

Then within about six to eight weeks, I can decide whether or not have the nipple area and the tattooing applied to the areola area since all that tissue was removed when I had the double mastectomy.

Monday, January 11, 2010 was the morning I returned to my family physician Dr. Kia's office. I haven't seen her since July 2009 when she gave me my cancer diagnosis.

It was a really good visit that included big hugs and questions from her as to what I actually went through; both pre- and post-op. Dr. Kia told me I need to increase my calcium intake from 600 mg to 1200 mg, and that I also need to start taking Evista, which is a medication for osteoporosis.

It seems I have osteoporosis in my lower back and my right hip. That makes me susceptible to a bone break, if I happen to fall.

We discussed a doctor for me to see for my ovaries. His name is Dr. Doug Idding. He actually does robotic surgery at Genesys Hospital. Something I probably will need to take care of within about six months or so. Because of the BRCA gene that causes ovarian cancer, I am at risk for that also. I also have a small fibroid tumor on my uterine wall, but it is very small and not cancerous.

Dr. Kia also discussed with me about getting my eyes examined (dilated) because of my Type 2 Diabetes. I am also required to get some blood work done to check my sugar and thyroid levels. I'll be doing all of this next week. I need to increase my glucotrol medication to 500 additional milligrams in the afternoon since my glucose levels seem to be a little too high in the evenings.

All in all, I feel rather normal and really good, even though my chassis seems to be deteriorating slightly. This is all due to age I'm sure.

It has been 19 days since my implant surgery, and I am wondering when I will start feeling like these implants are part of my body and not foreign objects that extend out from my chest. The size and shape are not too big, or exactly what I expected, but Dr. Pummill explained that when augmentation is done, the breasts actually are more cone shaped then when the implants are put into place. Since there is no tissue there when they are placed in, they actually are wider and a little flatter than augmentation.

Either way, I am just happy to have boobies again.

It's Monday, January 18, 2010, and it's another busy morning. After fasting yesterday, I headed to Dr. Kia's office and had blood drawn again to check my glucose levels and my thyroid.

Afterwards, I was able to enjoy breakfast with my better half. We don't get to do that very often, so it was a treat. Then Mike drove me to my 10:00 a.m. appointment with Dr. Pummill.

She will be giving me cream to apply on my scars. I don't know if it was an oversight or I just don't remember, but she explained to me that I would need another outpatient procedure to make a nipple on each of my breasts. After that has been done and I heal more, I will then be tattooed in the areola area.

At 1:00 p.m., I was supposed to head to a new ophthalmologist, recommended by Dr. Kia, for my annual diabetic eye exam. But because of Mike's time constraints and because we only have one vehicle at this time, I had to reschedule the appointment for Friday morning.

It will feel good to be able to go home and just relax a little this afternoon, so that I can prepare Mike's dinner for him before he needs to go to work.

It's now Monday, January 25, 2010, and the week started out with my daughter celebrating her 37th birthday. It hardly seems possible that so much time has passed since we brought her home. Time really has a way of flying by.

This morning the computer monitor finally "gave up the ghost," joining the printer that died last week. So, Mike, Chad, and I went computer shopping so that we could continue "business as usual" on the computer. Our next-door neighbor helped us out greatly by installing the new computer and spyware.

My doctor appointments have slowed down for a while. Thank goodness, because Mike and I are tired of all these co-pays. I know I will be receiving at least two to three more bills because of my recent visit to Dr. Kia, the ophthalmologist, and having blood drawn. Oh well. Guess I will just have to take it one bill at a time.

I am healing well and have run out of the scar cream samples that Dr. Pummill gave me at my last trip to her office. So, I will need to purchase a tube of Mediderm and a tube of Kelo-cote. I know the Kelo-cote will cost $25.00, but I have no idea how much the Mediderm runs. I have been taking the Evista for osteoporosis that Dr. Kia prescribed in the morning with my other meds, but I think I will start taking it in the afternoon with my Glucophage, as it seems to be making me a little nauseous in the mornings.

Otherwise, I have no real side effects with its usage. I am hoping it will help reverse the effects of the osteoporosis, or at least slow its progress down. I am starting to feel the slight signs of aging as each year passes, as I also found out that I have slight cataract starting in my left eye. Let's see that means I have Type 2 diabetes, some osteoporosis, I am a breast cancer survivor, and I am starting to get cataract. Sounds to me as if I need a new chassis.

I guess I will go into the living room for a little while and watch the evening news. I find myself being drawn to the news every night since the devastating earthquake in Haiti. My heart breaks for all those lost lives, for all the new orphans, and all the destroyed lives and homes as a result of the quake.

# February

Last week I went shopping for my first bra since my mastectomy surgery. It was really fun looking at all the styles, colors, and the pretty lace bras. I think I tried on about eight, making sure I had one that fit really well and was comfortable.

Finding something that comfortable and pretty was my goal. I was able to find two from the same manufacturer that I liked: one was beige and the other was taupe. I felt pretty and feminine. And I was even able to go up a size. Mike was very pleased and told me that I should go shopping another day and find a red one for Valentine's Day. I certainly don't need an excuse to go shopping again. That was fun!

Today is Saturday, the day before Valentine's Day, and Mike and I decided to take cards and a small gift to our daughter and grandchildren. After our visit, we went shopping at Kohl's for another bra or two for me.

While I was in the dressing room, I heard a voice outside the door say, "Grandpa. What are you doing here?" I thought the voice sounded familiar, so I cracked the door ajar and there was my granddaughter, Kristyn. I asked her what she was doing and she replied, "Shopping with a couple of my friends." I asked where her friends were and she said, "Hold on. I'll go get them." Off she scurried, returning within a couple of minutes with her friends, Nicole and Valerie.

They all came into my dressing room and I asked them if they wanted to see my battle scars. They were a little reluctant, but then they all said yes.

I showed them where the mastectomy had been done and was now replaced by my implants. The girls all said they were sorry I had to have the surgery, and they asked me if I had cancer in both breasts. I told them yes, and encouraged them to make sure they did self-examinations and to get their mammograms when they got older. They assured me they would and then they all helped me decide on which bras to purchase as I tried them on.

My granddaughter told me that my boobies looked really good, and that she was sorry that I had to endure what I did, but that she was really glad that I was OK. She then asked me if I would have lunch with her at Easter. Her friends went into another dressing room to try on their own undergarments while Kristyn stayed with me and asked if I would buy her some socks. We went to that area of the store and she found some socks that were on sale. We all went to the checkout area, and I gave her the bag. Kristyn told me her friends said "goodbye" and that they were really glad to have met me. She then said, "Grandma. You need to go into the junior department and buy yourself a cute pair of jeans." I told her I would do that another time. Then she gave Mike and I a hug, said she loved us, and hurried to meet up with her friends again.

I'm really glad I ran into my granddaughter today. It made my shopping experience even more fun, and it is always nice to see her and exchange hugs with her.

Today, in the middle of another snowstorm, I had an appointment with my plastic surgeon, Dr. Pummill. She once again reiterated that I am healing beautifully, that I am very symmetrical, and that the actual implants are softening up a bit more.

My next procedure, nipple reconstruction, is scheduled for March 24, 2010 at 7:30 a.m. I will be given general anesthesia, and the skin that is on top of the implant area will be stitched so that it resembles a small bump. The stitches will again dissolve and the bandages will need to stay in place for three to four days. It will be difficult to shower again for a couple of days, but I am almost finished with the actual reconstruction process. The only thing left to be done is the actual coloring (tattooing) in the areola area.

Dr. Pummill said that would probably be done two to three weeks after the nipple procedure. The good news is that this procedure and the coloring process will be covered by my insurance. It is hard to believe that only six months has passed since my initial diagnosis. The time has gone by relatively fast because of all the doctor's appointments, but I can actually see light at the end of the tunnel now.

I am feeling really good and people that know me say I have never looked healthier. They all tell me that my coloring is good and I look really happy. I've been blessed with a really wonderful team of doctors, as well as the Great Physician, looking after me. I will share more after the next procedure has been completed.

As my journey gets closer to its end, I want to get a little personal, and share a couple of important things with those of you just getting ready to embark on this journey; or those of you who may be in the midst of it already.

I want everyone being diagnosed to know that it is normal to be scared at the time when you first hear the news. I learned this very quickly on August 18, 2009. It is also very normal to wonder how you will look after having the surgery. After all, half of what our womanhood represents will be gone. Shopping for lingerie and swimsuits will be a different experience than what we are used to.

It is normal to experience fear when you have to share with your loved ones what you are experiencing as this dark disease attacks your body. It is also normal to wonder how this disease will affect your married life, as well as your sex life with your partner.

The only thing I can tell you, is gain as much knowledge as you can about this disease called cancer. Please make sure when you are given your initial cancer diagnosis that you seek out a franchised-trained breast surgeon. There is a world of difference between this kind of surgeon and a general surgeon.

Surround yourself with a surgeon that has your best interest and well being at heart. This is *your* life and *your* body, and you must be *your* own best advocate so that you can make good, sound, and informed choices. Create your own little team filled with excellent doctors who are up-to-date in their fields of specialty, and that take time to explain *every* aspect of what you will be experiencing.

Make yourself aware of any and all genetic testing that may be available to you. Take every advantage of sonograms, mammograms, and digital computer-generated MRI's at your disposal. Ask as many questions as you need to — make yourself knowledgeable.

This is *your* life and the quality of *your* life we're talking about.

Another important thing is to make sure you keep copies of all your tests, procedures, diagnosis reports, and go over each and every bill that comes your way. For example, after my nipple surgery, I received a bill for $5,000. I called Blue Cross Blue Shield of Michigan because I knew this should have been covered as part of my reconstruction. Sure enough, it had been coded as cosmetic surgery and not reconstructive surgery, so it will be covered.

While I was on the phone with BCBS, I also asked about my colorization process taking place on May 20, 2010 to make sure that is a covered procedure also. I was told that it was, and that I did not need to worry about receiving a bill for that. Mistakes do happen. That's why it's so important to look over every bill and statement you receive.

Remember, you might look different on the outside, but you will still be the same person on the inside. You will still be around to enjoy the sunshine, the changing of the seasons, walks on the bench, quiet nights at home with your loved ones, and just time in general.

Celebrate life!

Today is Wednesday, March 17, 2010 —
Happy St. Patty's Day!

This holiday celebrates half of my
heritage, as I am Irish, French Canadian,
and Hungarian.

Last night I received a phone call
from the surgery center where my nipple
reconstruction will take place next
Wednesday. The nurse reminded me of
the usual pre-op procedures: nothing to
eat after midnight the night before, no
medications except for my blood
pressure pill, no makeup, or jewelry. My
arrival time is 6:30 a.m., and my
procedure is at 7: 30 a.m. I am the first
one on the surgery docket again.

I am a little nervous about this
procedure, not sure why, but I think a
little might have to do with the fact that I
only have the colorization left to be done.
My journey is really near the end. It
hardly seems possible that six months
have actually gone by since my
diagnosis, and yet sometimes it seems
like an eternity.

I keep getting encouragement from loved ones, and get well or encouragement cards are still arriving, which helps to keep me motivated and upbeat.

Two days after the nipple reconstruction procedure, I'll have a post-op visit with Dr. Pummill. Then I only have to wait two weeks more until the colorization process is done in her office. At that time I will be whole again and look as normal as humanly possible. I hope I look as good as I feel when everything is said and done. Once again, I have complete confidence in my doctor and my Heavenly Father who still has His loving arms around me.

More to come after the procedure.

The next stage of the reconstruction process is now over. I arrived on time at the surgery center and was taken to the staging area. The nurse had trouble finding a working vein for the IV. I had to be poked in each hand, and the third poke took in my left arm. I got sick to my stomach and vomited a little, and my head and back got real sweaty, but I made it through.

Dr. Pummill was a little late arriving, but she greeted me and then marked me up with her pen, and off we went to the surgery room.

I did much better this time coming out of the anesthesia, so I was only there a total of four hours. I am now home resting, and I am experiencing a little pain (about two on a scale of one to ten) so I guess you could say I am doing well.

I will see Dr. Pummill at 8:30 a.m. this Friday, March 26, 2010. Then two weeks or so from now I will be going to her Grand Blanc office where she will numb both breasts with a local anesthetic and the colorization will take place. She told me it only takes about a half hour to an hour to complete.

By then I will look aesthetically pleasing and I will be anatomically correct. The whole breast cancer process and reconstruction will be over, and I will begin giving back to the American Cancer Society at their fundraising event in June, and the event in Holly in August.

I am very thankful and grateful to all who have brought me thus far and to all those family and friends who have supported me and prayed for me throughout this whole ordeal. Mostly I am thankful to my husband and children for their love and support, and thankful to the Lord who has watched over me.

I just returned from my post-op visit with Dr. Pummill. She said I look great. She told me that the nipples will seem a little large right now, but not to worry, they will shrink. I am to return for another visit in two weeks where she will examine me again to make sure that I am still healing all right.

In approximately six to eight weeks, the colorization will take place. I originally thought it would be in about two weeks, but it will give me more time to heal and to prepare for the final procedure.

Dr. Pummill said it is an easy procedure. I will be numbed with a shot and then she will perform her magic. She really is a wonderful plastic surgeon; very talented in what she does.

I have a come a long way and the journey is near its end. It feels really wonderful to be this close to being done. I look forward to the future and all that it will hold for Mike and I.

My second post-op appointment with Dr. Pummill was the day after Easter and it went well. At that time, she made my colorization appointment for May 20, 2010. That will be the last procedure I will experience since this whole journey started in August 2009. It hardly seems possible that this much time has passed, but I am very thankful it is near its end.

Just a little change of plans: I received a phone call from Dr. Pummill's office today requesting that my colorization process be moved up by one week. Dr. Pummill has a surgery planned on May 20, so it looks like I will be going in on May 13 instead. That's alright with me because when the process is finished, I will be back to normal. Or at least as normal as is physically possible. It seems really good to know that my journey is almost over.

I look forward to being able to share with others about what has happened to me, and I look forward to giving back at "Relay for Life" in June and the "Reunion with a Cause" fundraiser in Holly, Michigan in August.

Today I also received my first reimbursement check for $50 from my implant company. The check was sent because I filled out their survey. Each survey I fill out, and each yearly visit to my surgeon will allow me to receive another check.

Because I am the recipient of silicone implants, the company that produces them actually requires me to participate in an annual survey. I believe I will be involved in this for several years. I am also required to see my surgeon on the first, fourth, and ten-year anniversaries of my actual implant surgery.

I am very glad to be involved with a company that is so concerned with the well being of the patients who use their implants.

An interesting fact is that my implants are guaranteed for life. That warranty is better then most automobiles that I am aware of. I carry an identification card in my wallet that has the number of each implant, both right and left, for identification purposes. Guess I'll always be able to be identified if something awful happens. Who knew there was a funny side to breast cancer?

Last night I went to the Disabled American Veterans building with my husband for his monthly meeting; I am in the ladies auxiliary at the same location.

We discussed beautifying the grounds around the building, the upcoming Memorial Day Parade, our float that must be built, and the upcoming election of officers next month. After the meeting was closed, I asked if I could speak on a personal note.

I shared with the ladies that I was a recent breast cancer survivor, and that I would be participating in the "Relay for Life" sponsored by the American Cancer Society on the second weekend of June. I told them that I registered, that I was raising funds, and I would be participating in the survivor's lap. If anyone wanted to donate in my name, or sponsor the walk, they could do so. To my utter surprise, they voted to underwrite the total $200 amount that I was asked to raise. How totally awesome was that!

I was taken aback and humbled by their kindness. I called my sister-in-law as soon as I got back home to share the exciting news with her. She, along with her husband, had already donated $25. Between them and the ladies' auxiliary, I exceed my goal. I am hoping

141

to continue fundraising. I feel it is time for me to give back and I am totally excited about the process of raising more funds.

I also met two more ladies in the waiting room at Dr. Pummill's office. The first was going through the tissue expander process. She asked me about my current nipple reconstruction procedure and wanted to know if I was glad that I had undergone it.

The second lady was just in the process of being scheduled for a double mastectomy, as I had done, and wanted me to sit and talk with her. I know she was apprehensive, just as I was, but I reassured her and told her that she would love Dr. Pummill. She was experiencing the best in plastic surgery, and I wished her well in her journey. It was great to be able to share, and hopefully, I was able to help in small way. And so, each time I feel as if my journey is just about to end, I meet someone else going through this same experience, and it makes me realize my journey has just begun.

Today started with running errands. Mike and I went to Lowes' nursery to pick up some landscaping bricks.

We had started a flowerbed on the east side of the backyard and wanted to enclose the bed with bricks, just as we had done on the outside perimeter of the deck flowerbeds. I was also able to pick up some violas for two urns that I place in front of my garage entrance. Then we went to the grocery store to pick up an item that we'd paid for, but they had forgotten to pack with our other items. From there we had lunch together at Wendy's. Then it was on to K-Mart to pick up some potting soil for the plants that I bought. Finally, then it was home to start working in the yard.

After nine months of surgeries, healing, and reconstruction, it was really enjoyable for me to be able to plant flowers (which is my favorite thing to do) and to use the riding mower to mow the backyard. What fun! It really is great to be able to do the normal things that I truly enjoy again.

I am looking forward to my colorization process that will take place May 13, 2010. That is just before my 42$^{nd}$ wedding anniversary. My next project is the "Relay for Life" walk, sponsored by the American Cancer Society that will be held on June 12. I will be participating as a cancer survivor. Since Mike was my caregiver during all my procedures, he'll be going with me also. So far I have surpassed my $200 goal, and I am hoping to reach the $350 mark. We'll see. If you don't set a goal, then how will you know if you can reach it, right? So I might as well set it high.

I also received an e-mail from Dr. Gold today. She praised me for participating in the "Relay for Life" in June, and told me that it is an awesome program to be involved in. She said that the candlelight ceremony is very moving, and that the survivor's walk will mean a lot to me because I am one.

She also told me that she finished reading my journal, "One Lump, or Two," and that it needs to be a "book." According to her, I have a very good sense of humor, even in a difficult time, and that she feels the book will be very uplifting to others even though the topic is a difficult one. It was very good to have her opinion. She told me to enjoy my new "nipples" and to keep in touch with her. I plan on doing that very thing.

Mike had a doctor's appointment today, and I went with him. After he was finished, I told him I wanted to say hello to my family physician, Dr. Kia.

I explained to the receptionist that I was a recent breast cancer survivor and I just wanted to say hello. Dr. Kia came out into the waiting room and invited me into her office.

She told me that I looked great and asked me how everything was going. I told her I was to have my colorization process on May 13, and that I had just had my nipple construction about four and a half weeks ago. I told her I was a little nervous, but her comment was, "You'll do great."

She told me that she had kept the letter I sent her thanking her for her kindness to me, and for recommending such good surgeons to me.

She told me that it wasn't just the surgeons that helped my healing process, it was me! She said that she was very proud of me because of my positive spirit and my involvement in every aspect of my treatment. She also said she talks about me to her other patients and explains to them how important their mammograms are.

She tells them that I had my physicals, pap smears, and mammograms every year faithfully, and yet, I was still diagnosed with double breast cancer.

I told her that I was participating in the Grand Blanc "Relay for Life" the second Saturday of June. She asked where it would be held and said that she might just show up with her little daughter. I told her that would be great, and that I hoped I would see her there.

I also told her about my journal, and she said she definitely wanted to read it. I told her I was trying to get it published as an encouragement for others. She told me that would be great, and was proud that I wanted to share.

She gave me a great big hug and told me that she loved me, and that I was an awesome patient. I told her that I just did what I had to do, but that I had a lot of prayers and support from friends and loved ones to help me along the way.

I am really glad that I stopped in to see Dr. Kia. She really made me feel great today.

This morning, May 13, 2010, was the day that I had my last procedure since being diagnosed with breast cancer back in August 2009. It feels very good to be finally finished.

The colorization process took only about 45 minutes. I was taken back into the procedure room at Dr. Pummill's office and numbed up. That was the worst part of the procedure, although, it really wasn't too bad. After the first initial sting of the needle, I actually felt just a little twinge now and then.

Dr. Pummill then marked me where she wanted to tattoo the area and talked to me about mixing the pigment. We decided on a pinkish brown. I asked Dr. Pummill since I was doing a custom color, could she add some gold metallic to give me some bling. She just laughed and told me I was really funny.

She expressed to me how great I looked and that I was inspiring to her and her staff because of the way I handled everything I had to go through. I told her that if I hadn't had such a good team of doctors and support from those I love and friends that I probably wouldn't have done so well. Her reply was that I underestimate myself and that I don't give myself enough credit.

I took Dr. Pummill's picture, as well as those of Becky and Kristen, her office assistants. After some big hugs to everyone I left the office.

I am now anatomically correct and feel very, very lucky and so, this part of my journey ends.

I would like to end my journal talking about my first experience with the "Relay for Life." The event was held at Grand Blanc High School on June 12, 2010.

Mike and I arrived at 9:20 a.m., and walked around a bit waiting for the opening ceremony at 10:00 a.m. At the opening ceremony, all the teams were front and center, and we all read the cancer society pledge. With that reading, my eyes teared up and I felt more emotional than I thought I would.

I went home for a while to eat lunch with my husband and relax a bit. We returned to the grounds for a 2:00 p.m. fight back ceremony, where those that wanted to help "fight back" made pledges not to smoke, to get more exercise, to eat healthier, and to promote cancer information.

At 5:50 p.m., all the survivors and their caregivers were asked to come near the stage and we were instructed about the survivor lap, where we would all make one lap around the track together, then the caregivers would make one lap, and then return with us.

At that time, all the survivors in purple shirts, with purple balloons were asked to let their balloons go at once.

All you could see was this purple mass of balloons rising into the heavens. Another symbolic gesture that we were survivors, and that we were still here. A neighbor of mine, also a survivor, was my buddy all through the day. She grabbed my arm and we took the survivor laps together. Again the tears welled up in my eyes. Two precious little boys about six or seven years of age were cheering,

"You made it. Good job. You're still here." It was very touching because I realized that they were cheering for me, and they didn't even know me.

After the survivor and caregiver laps, we were asked to go into the registration tent where we were served a dinner of salad, lasagna, buffalo wild wings, pasta salad, and birthday cake. The birthday cake represented all the birthdays ahead of us as survivors. There was also a group of young children that sang "Happy Birthday" to all of us before we ate dinner, and they passed out birthday cards to all of us.

Once we ate, Mike and I went home to relax a little again before the candlelight ceremony. All the luminaries were lit and we all did laps around the track again in complete silence, and with the candles in our hands. There were also Tiki torches lit all along Saginaw Avenue. These luminaries and torches represented all the cancer patients that did not make it. There was a single bagpiper playing as we walked around the track several times in honor of those that had passed. Again, a very tearful and touching moment for me.

The ceremonies ended with a young lady singing, "God is Faithful to Me."

Mike and I departed after hugs and goodbyes to my "survivor buddy" and her family. It was a long day and very hot, but I am very thankful that I participated and that my husband was able to be with me again for this important ceremony.

It was also nice to be able to clap for him and cheer him on as he did his caregiver lap in honor of me.

Through an e-mail the next day, I found out that $96,000 was raised the day of the relay, and another $1,800 was brought in through e-mails and phone calls.

It was my first cancer walk, but I think all in all, it was a great success.

# Epilogue

It hardly seems possible that ten months have passed since my cancer diagnosis, and a lot has transpired since this time. I had my double mastectomy, my tissue expander procedure, my implant surgery, my nipple construction, and now my colorization process.

I am anatomically correct and pretty much back to normal now. I feel that I owe my "A" team of doctors a heartfelt "thank you" for their expertise and care that they favored upon me.

I also owe much love and gratitude to my husband and my family for their support and care during my healing process and recuperation.

I thank my next-door neighbors for their generous gifts of food, cards, and flowers.

I am also very thankful to God above for watching over me and answered prayers that were offered up for me by friends, those I have never met, and loved ones. I know my faith has helped see me through this difficult time.

I feel that I have been blessed, and that the writing of this journal has been very cathartic for me. I was able to express myself on paper in a way that I know I could not have done any other way.

So, as this journey reaches its final writings, I hope that in some small way this journal may give hope and encouragement to others, because there is hope. I am living proof of that fact. As long as there is life, there *is* hope.

Approximately 1 in 8 women will hear, "You have breast cancer." When Linda Sadler heard those words on August 18, 2009, her life did changed direction forever.

Keeping a journal to document every twist and turn, Linda takes the reader on a honest journey — from her initial diagnosis, to her decision to have a double mastectomy, and her healing process.

Using humor to diffuse the dark shadows that come with this disease, Linda candidly shares what she discovered about breast cancer, and more importantly the strength and hope she found deep within her to face it head on and win.

For more information from this author and others like her, go to www.RochesterMedia.com